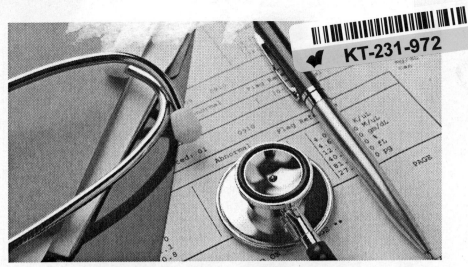

Succeeding in the GPST Stage 3 Selection Centre

Practice scenarios for GPST/ GPVTS Stage 3 assessments

Gayathri Rabindra, Nicole Corriette, Hamed Khan, Chirag Mehta & Matt Green

Second Edition

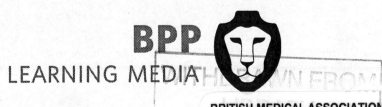

First edition 2009
Second edition November 2011

ISBN 9781 4453 8161 9
Previous ISBN 9781 9068 3903 1
e-ISBN 9781 4453 8583 9

British Library Cataloguing-in-Publication Data
A catalogue record for this book is available from
the British Library

Published by
BPP Learning Media Ltd
BPP House, Aldine Place
London W12 8AA

www.bpp.com/health

Typeset by Replika Press Pvt Ltd, India
Printed in the United Kingdom

Your learning materials, published by BPP
Learning Media Ltd, are printed on paper
sourced from sustainable, managed forests.

The views expressed in this book are those of
BPP Learning Media and not those of the NHS.
BPP Learning Media are in no way associated
with or endorsed by the NHS.

The contents of this book are intended as a guide
and not professional advice. Although every effort
has been made to ensure that the contents of
this book are correct at the time of going to
press, BPP Learning Media, the Editor and the
Author make no warranty that the information
in this book is accurate or complete and accept
no liability for any loss or damage suffered by
any person acting or refraining from acting as
a result of the material in this book.

Every effort has been made to contact the
copyright holders of any material reproduced
within this publication. If any have been
inadvertently overlooked, BPP Learning Media
will be pleased to make the appropriate credits
in any subsequent reprints or editions.

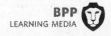

Contents

About the Publisher   *vi*
Free Companion Material   *vii*
About the Authors   *viii*
Acknowledgements   *x*

Chapter 1   **Introduction**   **1**
     Stage 1   2
     Stage 2   2
     Stage 3   3
     Stage 4   3
     Advice for the assessment   4

Chapter 2   **Important topics in General Practice**   **7**
     Audit   8
     Summary care record (national patient record database)   8
     Choose and Book (CaB)   9
     Out of Hours   9
     Practice Based Commissioning   9
     GPs with a Special Interest (GPSI, GPwSI)   9
     Significant Event Analysis   10
     General Medical Services Contract   10
     Quality and Outcomes Framework (QoF)   10
     National Institute for Health and Clinical Excellence (NICE)   11
     A day in the life of a GP   11
     GMC guidance   12
     Patient safety   12
     Confidentiality   13
     Confidentiality and children   14
     Child Protection issues   15
     Working with patients   16
     Guidance on accepting gifts from patients   16
     Arranging cover   17

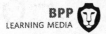

Contents

Chapter 3 Simulated exercises   19

Introduction   20
    What do the simulated exercises involve?   20
    Format of the simulated exercises   21
    Common topics in the simulated exercises   22
    Assessment criteria for the simulated exercises   23
    Mark scheme for the simulated exercises   25
General practice consultations versus hospital
based clerkings   28
Concepts for the simulated exercises   30
Skills required for the consultation   34
General tips for the simulated exercises   39
Suggested approach to the simulated exercises   47
Suggested approach to the consultation   47
Special scenarios   68
    Breaking bad news   68
    Dealing with the angry or upset patient, relative or
    colleague   70
    How to cope when things go wrong   71
Practice simulated exercises   72
    Structure of the practice consultations in this book   73
    How to give feedback   74
    Proposed mark scheme   75
    Practise to time   79
    Practise, practise, practise   80
Mock Consultation 1   81
Mock Consultation 2   99
Mock Consultation 3   117
Mock Consultation 4   135
Mock Consultation 5   153
Mock Consultation 6   173
Mock Consultation 7   187
Mock Consultation 8   201
Mock Consultation 9   213
Mock Consultation 10   225

Chapter 4 The prioritisation exercise   239

    The format of the prioritisation exercise   241
    Example prioritisation exercise: Scenario 1   242
    National Person Specification criteria
    assessed in the prioritisation exercise   244

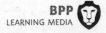

How are you marked? 251

The key to succeeding in the prioritisation cxercise 252

How to approach the exercise systematically 254

Reflection question 262

Answering the reflection question 262

Before the day 264

On the day 265

Worked example – Scenario 1 267

Practice Scenario 2 288

Practice Scenario 3 305

Practice Scenario 4 320

Practice Scenario 5 334

Practice Scenario 6 348

Practice Scenario 7 352

Practice Scenario 8 356

Practice Scenario 9 361

Practice Scenario 10 366

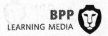

About the Publisher

BPP Learning Media is dedicated to supporting aspiring professionals with top quality learning material. BPP Learning Media's commitment to success is shown by our record of quality, innovation and market leadership in paper-based and e-learning materials. BPP Learning Media's study materials are written by professionally-qualified specialists who know from personal experience the importance of top quality materials for success.

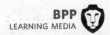

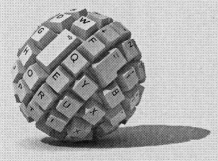

Free Companion Material

Readers can access blank mark schemes, to use with the exercises in this book, for free online.

To access the above companion material please visit **www.bpp.com/freehealthresources**

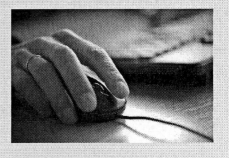

About the Authors

Nicole Corriette, MBBS (Hons) (London) BSc (Hons) (London) MRCGP DFSRH DRCOG DCH

After winning numerous awards at UCL Nicole completed her MRCGP with a distinction overall and was nominated for the Fraser Rose medal by the RCGP. She is currently a partner in a large practice and delivers GPST preparation courses.

Matt Green, BSc (Hons) MPhil

After completing his BSc in Biochemistry Matt went on to complete an MPhil at the Royal Marsden Hospital in London. This involved working closely with medical professionals on a number of projects developing novel drugs for the treatment of ovarian cancer. Since 2005 Matt has been supporting doctors to progress their career through providing application and interview advice together with helping doctors to develop their non-clinical skills including leadership, management, teaching and communication.

Hamed Khan, MBBS (London)

Hamed Khan graduated in 2006 from Barts and The London Medical School. After completing an Academic Medical Education Foundation Programme, he started a GP Vocational Training Scheme in South London. He has extensive experience of teaching medical undergraduates, and has published in various journals. Currently he is the Lead for Education on the London Deanery GP Trainee Committee.

Chirag Mehta, MBChB, MRCGP, DRCOG, DFSRH, Cert MedEd

Chirag Mehta is currently a salaried GP working in the West Midlands Deanery and obtained his MRCGP in 2011. He has a keen interest in medical education and is currently doing his diploma in medical education at Keele University.

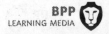

Gayathri Rabindra, MBBS (London) MA (Cantab.)

Gayathri Rabindra studied pre-clinical medicine at Cambridge University and completed her medical degree at Royal Free and University College Medical School. She is currently a GPST1 on the Sidcup Vocational Training Scheme, having successfully gained a place in the London Deanery.

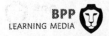

Acknowledgements

I would like to thank Dean Williams for all his help and support in writing this book. I would also like to thank Matt Green for giving me the opportunity to be part of the BPP Learning Media team.

Nicole Corriette

I would like to thank the hard efforts of the other contributing authors in helping to make this book a reality.

Matt Green

Thank you to BPP Learning Media for giving me the opportunity to write this book. I am very grateful to Anita Shah, Natalie Ng Man Sun and Tom Nolan, for their comments and tips. Thanks to my mum for her insights about the life of a GP, and for her unrelenting love and support.

Gayathri Rabindra

For my parents Khalid and Hajrah, and their ever-present support, encouragement and advice. I would also like to thank Dev Malhotra and John Chan for their valuable contributions.

Hamed Khan

I would like to thank Matt Green and BPP Learning Media for allowing me to contribute to this book.

Chirag Mehta

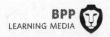

Chapter 1
Introduction

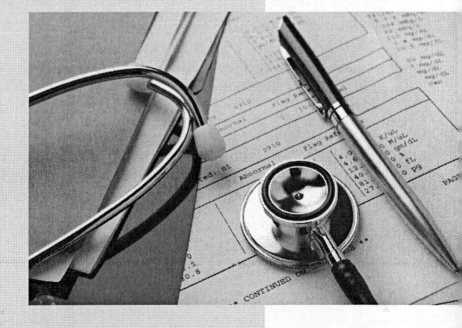

Introduction

Welcome to the BPP Learning Media GPST Stage 3 Preparation book, and well done on choosing General Practice as the career on which to set your sights. To gain the full benefit from this book you can visit www.bpp.com/freehealthresources to download blank mark schemes to use with each of the exercises. Despite all the changes in the NHS, General Practice has retained its core values which make it a unique and attractive career path. Adopting a holistic approach to patients, continuity of care, having control of your working environment and the huge variety offered by this speciality are just some of its attractions. Based on this it has become a very competitive speciality, with more and more trainees applying each year. The current GP recruitment process has been running for a number of years now and has been proven to be robust and fair. There are a number of stages involved. This allows a more complete assessment of candidates' suitability to General Practice than a single exam, application or interview.

There are four stages to the application process:

Stage 1
An online application that checks whether you are eligible for GP training. Everyone who is eligible is invited to the next stage.

Stage 2
An assessment which is conducted under invigilated conditions, and takes place at various centres around the country. It consists of two papers:

Paper 1: Clinical Problem Solving. This tests your ability to apply clinical knowledge to various scenarios. It is designed to be appropriate to the knowledge-base of a Foundation Year 2 doctor.

Paper 2: Professional Dilemmas. This tests your professional attributes and whether you are able to deal with various clinical and non-clinical scenarios in an appropriate way (for more details of our Stage 2 book see the inside back cover of this book).

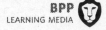

Those with the highest scores will be invited to attend the Stage 3 assessment at their first choice deanery. Depending on the availability of places and your national ranking, you could be allocated to an assessment at your second or third choice deanery.

Stage 3

A practical assessment, in which candidates are assessed against the National Person Specification. There are two parts to the assessment:

- Simulation Exercise (involving three different role-plays with an actor-patient)
- Written Prioritisation Task

Stage 4

This is the allocation and acceptance of places. If candidates are not offered a place at their first choice deanery, they may be offered a job at another deanery, depending on scores and availability of places.

Candidates are assessed against the National Person Specification. Throughout the application process, the competencies that are assessed are:

Clinical Skills
- This is mainly application of clinical knowledge.

Personal Skills
- Empathy and Sensitivity: This is crucial to any part of medicine: the ability to take other people's perspectives into account and to treat people with a non-judgemental approach.
- Communication Skills: You must be able to adapt to different patients and communicate with people in different situations.
- Conceptual Thinking and Problem Solving: The assessments are not looking for the most knowledgeable doctors, but rather those who have the ability to apply that knowledge in various situations.

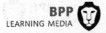

- Coping with Pressure. You must be able to recognise your own limitations and have strategies to cope with these, including seeking help from others.
- Organisation and Planning.
- Managing Others and Team Involvement.

Probity

- Professional Integrity. This is having the ability to take responsibility, as well as having respect for others.

Commitment to Speciality

- Learning and Personal Development. It is important to be able to reflect on one's experiences and learn from them, and continuously update skills and knowledge.

For more information visit the GP Recruitment website: www.gprecruitment.org.uk. Ensure that you regularly check this website for updates and assessment information. It includes examples of the exercises and important information about what is expected from candidates.

The Stage 3 assessment does well at assessing ability, but preparation and practice can help to ensure that your ability and aptitude shows through. It is not a test of knowledge as such, but rather consists of various practical exercises so there is no substitute for practising scenarios. Practising scenarios allows you to find the right frame of mind and to think about the competencies on which you are being tested. Some of the exercises, such as the simulated patient consultation, may be second nature as it is what we all do in our day-to-day lives. It is worth thinking about the techniques you use with patients and improving them to ensure you are adopting a patient-centred approach, and are always treating the patient with respect.

Advice for the assessment

Do make sure you read and re-read the information sent to you (usually by email). Some deaneries have a range of dates and you may be able to choose which date and time you attend. Try and do this as soon as possible, as popular deaneries fill up quickly and

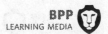

you might not be able to book a time convenient to you. Check the date, time and location, and plan your route in advance. The assessment usually runs over half a day, either the morning or afternoon. Around the time of the assessments there are bound to be rumours about what scenarios have already been used. It can be easy to get worried and stressed about what you hear, or feel disadvantaged if you are one of the first to attend the assessment. Don't worry about this, as the assessment is testing core attributes of candidates, as opposed to knowledge. Prior knowledge of the scenarios is unlikely to be useful.

What should you wear? It's important that you are comfortable in whatever you choose, but do make sure you are smart. Some people wear suits, whereas others wear smart work clothes. Do take a watch with you, as this will help in timing the tasks.

When you arrive at the selection centre, you will be given a candidate number and will find out in what order you will be doing the exercises. There will be someone to take your photos in candidate order; this is to ensure that the right person is attending the assessment, and to act as a trigger for the assessors to remember you during their discussions at the end of the day. There will be a waiting area for candidates with refreshments. This would be a good opportunity to introduce yourself to the other candidates who will be doing the group discussion with you. This will enable you all to be more relaxed during the exercise. Do make sure you are polite to everybody; even though you are not technically being assessed outside the exercises it doesn't hurt to make a good impression.

You will be required to bring various documents with you on the day. Don't leave this to the last minute as there are some things, such as references, which require preparation. Check the email and website for exactly what is required. Sometimes the original and a copy are required. The documentation usually required are listed below:

- A copy of the invitation email
- Passport
- Evidence of entitlement to work in the UK if you are not a UK or EU national

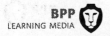

- GMC certificate
- Driving licence, or a letter stating how you will attend home visits if you cannot drive
- References. Usually three are required, and there may be a particular form that the referees are required to fill in. This can take some effort and time, so do start obtaining these as early as possible
- Degree certificate
- Evidence of Foundation Competencies. If you are a foundation doctor, your FY1 competencies certificate and a letter from your educational supervisor stating that you are expected to achieve FY2 competencies will suffice. Non-foundation doctors will need to take evidence stating that they have achieved the equivalent competencies. See the GP Recruitment website for details
- IELTS (Evidence of English Language knowledge) if appropriate
- Job selection form. Some selection centres will send you a form in advance, asking you to rank the various programmes in the deanery. This is important to do in advance, to give you the chance to research the various areas so you know what you're letting yourself in for. It is very unlikely that you will be able to change the location of your job once you have been offered one, and if you end up in Land's End when you wanted London, then you have nobody to blame but yourself!

In this book there is a chapter on each of the assessments you will encounter in Stage 3. The basic principles for each will be discussed and the approaches that can be taken. There are examples for you to practise under timed-conditions which we suggest you do with peers who are also undertaking the assessment. Be honest with each other, reflect on your attempts and keep a National Person Specification close to hand. The more you act on feedback and improve, the better you will be on the day.

Good luck!

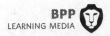

Chapter 2

Important topics in General Practice

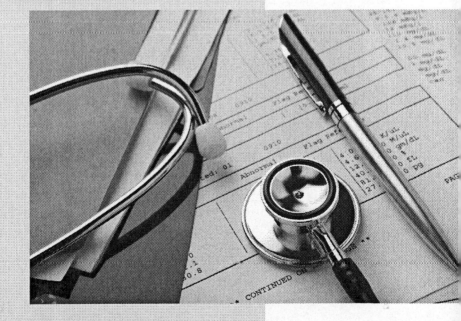

Important topics in General Practice

Succeeding in the Stage 3 assessment requires a good understanding of the role of a GP, their day to day practice and the organisation of primary care. This chapter contains brief explanations of some of the key aspects of General Practice, and a discussion of some GMC guidance of which to be aware for the assessment.

Audit

Clinical audit is a process which reviews current clinical practice against a defined set of standards. If it is found that practice is sub-standard, then recommendations should be made and changes implemented to improve practice. Audit doesn't stop there; it's important to repeat the audit to see whether these changes have had the desired effect. You can use audit to evaluate your own practice or that of your department, surgery or hospital.

Clinical audit is an important part of **clinical governance**. This is the process of ensuring that NHS organisations continually improve the quality of their services, and maintain high standards of care.

This can be achieved through audit, education and training, learning from near misses and significant events, ensuring that patient's views are taken into account, and implementing guidelines and policies.

Summary care record (national patient record database)

This is an initiative which would allow patient records to be stored in one place. It is part of the NHS programme 'Connecting for Health' and aims to allow easier access to patient records and thus allow clinicians to obtain definitive information regarding patients. At present, there is nothing to allow a hospital to obtain access to the records of a patient that are held in another hospital, and patient care suffers for this. With this system, as long as the records are secure and confidentiality maintained, then a big hurdle in healthcare could be removed.

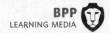

Choose and Book (CaB)

In the past, when GPs made referrals for patients to see a specialist in hospital, patients had to wait to hear about their appointment date and had no choice as to when this was. With 'Choose and Book', when the decision for referral has been made, the GP can log onto a system which will allow the patient to see what appointments are available in all the nearby hospitals. From these they can pick a slot which suits them. This should decrease the number of missed appointments and allows patients to choose where and when they have their appointment. However it takes up time and in a short GP consultation this can be a problem.

Out of Hours

Many GPs have opted out of providing night and weekend care, and therefore the Primary Care Trust takes over the responsibility of providing out of hours care. They employ people to provide cover. Recently, the government has stipulated that GP surgeries should increase access to patients outside of normal working hours. Not all practices have extended their opening hours, but some are now open for a few hours on Saturdays and longer into the evenings during the week.

Practice Based Commissioning

As services in the community can often be provided at a cheaper rate than in secondary care, Practice Based Commissioning (PBC) allows GP practices to commission or provide services for their local communities. The PCT supports GP practices (often groups of practices) in 'buying in' services for their patients based on cost and quality of care.

GPs with a Special Interest (GPSI, GPwSI)

These are GPs with additional training in a specific clinical area (for example, cardiology or dermatology) who are able to take referrals and see patients that would otherwise have been referred to hospitals. They can therefore decrease demand for secondary care services which are usually far more expensive than primary care. They can also provide an enhanced service for specific conditions or patient groups.

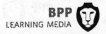

Significant Event Analysis

A Significant Event Analysis (SEA) looks at an individual case or event that led to a significant outcome in detail. This allows people to learn from the case, to see whether anything could have been done differently, and can highlight system failures which can be improved to prevent a similar incident occurring.

General Medical Services Contract

This is the contract between general practices and primary care organisations to deliver primary care services to their local communities. The funding that the practice receives depends on various factors. The more patients that are registered with the practice the more money the practice generates. Additional income can be obtained by offering additional services, such as minor surgery or care of patients with substance abuse. In addition, funding is provided through the Quality and Outcomes Framework.

Quality and Outcomes Framework (QoF)

This was introduced in April 2004 as a financial incentive for GP practices to provide higher standards of care. Points are available for clinical and non-clinical aspects of care, and the higher the number of points achieved, the more money that the practice receives.

The main domains are:

- **Clinical** standards linked to the care of patients suffering from chronic diseases, for example, cardiovascular disease and COPD
- **Organisational** standards relating to records and information, communicating with patients, education and training, medicines management and clinical and practice management
- **Additional services**, covering cervical screening, child health surveillance, maternity services and contraceptive services
- **Patient experience**, based on patient surveys and length of consultations

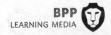

National Institute for Health and Clinical Excellence (NICE)

NICE is an independent organisation and is responsible for providing national guidance on the management of medical conditions. They look at evidence and evaluate the cost-effectiveness of treatments.

A day in the life of a GP

The work of a GP is varied and unpredictable, and these are some of the reasons why it is so enjoyable. Let us describe a typical day of a GP partner.

As soon as you arrive at work you check through emails which may include the latest NICE guidelines or the minutes of the last practice meeting. Before morning surgery you might quickly check through some blood results and letters from the hospital, making a note of anything that will require chasing up later.

You start your morning surgery and see 15 patients with routine appointments plus a number of emergency appointments as well. There might be a couple of patients with chronic problems that take a while to sort out, but if you're lucky a few quick coughs and colds might help you make up the time. Morning surgery finishes around midday. You might have some telephone consultations to make and repeat prescriptions to sign off before you grab some lunch.

A variety of things happen during your lunch break depending on the day of the week: a meeting with the Practice Manager to discuss issues affecting the practice, staff, or finances; postgraduate meetings at the nearby hospital; a primary care multidisciplinary meeting; or the weekly Practice meeting.

Every clinical session creates a mountain of paperwork such as referral letters and insurance reports, so you'll probably try to fit some of this in before afternoon surgery. You might not have a chance though, as there is usually a home visit or two to make. At around 3 o'clock afternoon surgery begins, with another 10–15 patients to see. For those who are keen, rather than going home after a long day's work, it's straight on to an out-of-hours GP session.

Dr K Rabindra-Anandh,
GP Partner, Romford

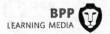

GMC guidance

It is important to ensure that you are familiar with the GMC's guidance for doctors. Themes relating to this can come up in any of the two tasks, and will be useful during medical practice.

Patient safety

The GMC guide *Good Medical Practice* clearly states that as a doctor, you must make patient safety a priority:

> *If you have good reason to think that patient safety is or may be seriously compromised by inadequate premises, equipment, or other resources, policies or systems, you should put the matter right if that is possible. In all other cases you should draw the matter to the attention of your employing or contracting body. If they do not take adequate action, you should take independent advice on how to take the matter further. You must record your concerns and the steps you have taken to try to resolve them.*

If there is any immediate or potential risk to patients, then action must be taken to protect them. In the prioritisation task, situations where patient safety is compromised must be dealt with first and as a matter of urgency. It is also pertinent in situations where there is an 'underperforming colleague'. If there is any risk to patients if this colleague continues to work (for example, if he/she is drunk) then you must take steps to ensure that patients are safeguarded. The urgency of your actions would depend on the actual risk to patients. This is described in paragraphs 43–45 of *Good Medical Practice*:

> *You must protect patients from risk of harm posed by another colleague's conduct, performance or health. The safety of patients must come first at all times. If you have concerns that a colleague may not be fit to practise, you must take appropriate steps without delay, so that the concerns are investigated and patients are protected where necessary. This means you must give an honest explanation of your concerns to an appropriate person from your employing or contracting body, and follow their procedures.*

> *If there are no appropriate local systems, or local systems do not resolve the problem, and you are still concerned about the safety*

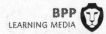

of patients, you should inform the relevant regulatory body. If you are not sure what to do, discuss your concerns with an impartial colleague or contact your defence body, a professional organisation, or the GMC for advice.

As detailed above, if you cannot deal with the matter yourself you should involve an appropriate senior colleague, such as a Registrar, Partner or Consultant – they may have more experience in this area. As well as safeguarding patients, ensure that your underperforming colleague has sufficient support to help them deal with their problems.

Confidentiality

The doctor–patient relationship is a sacred one, and confidentiality should be maintained at all times. However, there may be some situations where confidentiality must be broken, for example, to safeguard the safety of others. If you feel that this is necessary, then you must inform the patient that you are going to do so.

The GMC has guidance about when it is acceptable to breach confidentiality:

- If the patient consents to disclosure of information.
- If disclosure of information is required by law, for example with notifiable diseases. Patients should be informed about the disclosure but their consent is not required.
- If a judge or presiding officer of a court orders you to disclose information. However, you must not disclose information to solicitors, police officers or officers of a court without the patient's consent.
- If the disclosure is in the public interest. That is, if the benefits of the disclosure to an individual or society outweigh the public and the patient's interest in keeping the information confidential.

In all cases where you consider disclosing information without consent from the patient, you must weigh the possible harm (both to the patient, and the overall trust between doctors and patients) against the benefits which are likely to arise from the release of information.

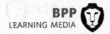

Wherever possible, it is still advisable to inform the patient that you are planning to disclose the information.

An example where it is acceptable to break confidentiality would be when a patient is driving against medical advice, for example after a fit. This is something that can come up in the patient consultation task, where you would be required to advise a patient of the risks of driving when they have had a fit, and the guidance about this.

The GMC states that *'The DVLA is legally responsible for deciding if a person is medically unfit to drive. The Agency needs to know when driving licence holders have a condition which may now, or in the future, affect their safety as a driver.'*

In the first instance, you should make sure that the patient in question understands that their condition can impair their ability to drive. In situations where they are unable to understand this information, for example in patients with dementia, then you should inform the DVLA immediately. With competent patients you should also explain to them that they have a legal duty to inform the DVLA. If they continue to drive, you must make a reasonable effort to persuade them to stop. This may include discussing with their next of kin if they consent to this. However, if you cannot persuade them to stop, or there is evidence that they are continuing to drive, then you should disclose relevant medical information to the medical adviser at the DVLA. Before you do this, you should advise the patient that you are doing so, and afterwards, write to the patient informing them that disclosure has been made.

In summary, if a patient is unfit to drive, you must make every effort to persuade them to inform the DVLA, but if they will not, then it is in the public's interest for you to break confidentiality in these cases. A case such as this can present itself during the patient consultation task, so ensure that you are familiar with the guidance.

Confidentiality and children

The same duties of confidentiality apply for adults as for children. Therefore, if you need to share information about a child with others, you would need their consent. However, this requires

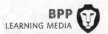

assessment of the capacity of the child in question. To assess capacity in children is the same as you would for adults, i.e. are they able to understand, believe and retain information so that they can understand the nature, risks and benefits of having a treatment, as well as the consequences of not having the treatment.

However, if it is deemed that the child lacks capacity, and they decline for you to share the information (for example, with a legal guardian who can consent for them), then the GMC offers the following guidance:

> You should usually try to persuade the child to involve a parent in such circumstances. If they refuse and you consider it is necessary in the child's best interests for the information to be shared (for example, to enable a parent to make an important decision, or to provide proper care for the child), you can disclose information to parents or appropriate authorities. You should record your discussions and reasons for sharing the information.

As is the case with adults, confidentiality can also be broken if there is an overriding public interest or disclosure of information is required by law.

Child Protection issues

Confidentiality can be broken if there are any concerns about a child's welfare, for example if you are concerned that a child is being abused by their parents. If the child is resistant to you disclosing information, then you must try your best to help them understand the benefits of sharing information. However, if any delay in sharing information would lead to an increased risk to the child or other children you must act swiftly. In the example of child abuse, social services would normally be the first port of call, however this would depend on your local policies.

Another issue is that of under-aged sexual intercourse. In these situations, you must judge whether the child is competent, and able to consent, while understanding the implications. However, anyone under the age of thirteen are considered by law to be unable to consent to sex, and thus sex with someone under the age of thirteen is considered rape. Therefore social services and

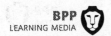

the police would have to be informed in these cases. If you have any suspicion that the sexual activity is forced upon the child, or if you suspect that the young person's sexual partner is abusing a position of trust, then this would also warrant discussion with social services.

Working with patients

It is imperative throughout your medical practice that you treat patients with dignity and listen considerately to their concerns. The GMC states that doctors should work in partnership with their patients; gone are the days where doctors are taught to adopt a paternalistic approach with patients. Instead you should *'respect patients' right to reach decisions with you about their treatment and care'*. Therefore, it is important that you give patients all the information and should work with them to come to a decision, rather than dictate to them what to do.

Consultations with patients are much more than just coming to a diagnosis. It is important to elicit their ideas, concerns and expectations (ICE). The insight you gain from this knowledge can help enormously with treatment, because if you can understand the situation from the patient's perspective, you will be able to help them deal with their condition. For example, you might see a patient with cough and cold symptoms. After assessing them you are confident that there are no signs of a chest infection you may be happy to simply dismiss the patient from the room. However, the patient may have been expecting antibiotics and will leave the room angry and dissatisfied if they do not understand the situation, as you have not elicited their expectations. Or they might be worried that they have cancer as their mother died from the same illness recently, but if you don't ask them what they think it is, then you will not be able to reassure them that they do not have cancer.

Guidance on accepting gifts from patients

Patients in hospital and in the community often give presents to their doctors, such as chocolates to express their gratitude for help with their treatment. But what is the guidance on this? The GMC states that:

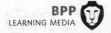

You must not encourage patients to give, lend or bequeath money or gifts that will directly or indirectly benefit you.

You must not put pressure on patients or their families to make donations to other people or organisations.

We should not encourage patients to give you gifts, but what if they were to give you a gift, should you accept it? In general, you would need to look at whether the gift is appropriate, for example, a box of chocolates after a ward stay is more reasonable than giving £200 to a particular doctor. Scenarios involving this situation could come up in any part of the assessment. Each situation would need to be analysed individually. It is important to ascertain whether the patient thinks they are obliged to give the present in order to receive good quality healthcare, and you must make sure that they realise that this is not the case. If the concern is a colleague accepting gifts, then the facts would need to be ascertained to find out whether they are coercing the patient to do so. If you decline a gift that seems inappropriate, do so sensitively and explain to the patient your reasons for doing so.

Arranging cover

Some parts of the Stage 3 assessment may involve issues of handover and cover, for example, going off duty when there is nobody to hand over to. The main point here is to ensure that patient safety is not put at risk. Therefore if your shift has ended but the next doctor has not arrived then you must wait until you can hand over. If you feel patient safety is at risk for any reason, for example by there not being enough doctors on the ward due to illness, then it would be worth saying that you would inform appropriate people to ensure that this is rectified, such as your Consultant or the department lead so that locum cover can be arranged.

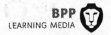

Chapter 3
Simulated exercises

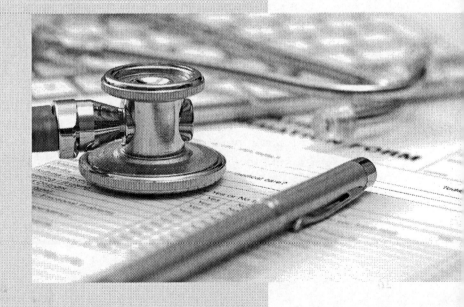

Simulated exercises

Introduction

The simulated exercise is literally what it says: an exercise that involves simulating a consultation in three different scenarios – a patient, a family member or carer and a colleague. It is designed to assess your interpersonal and communication skills, and not your clinical knowledge, as this has already been assessed in Stage 2 of the assessment. Therefore, the emphasis is much more on how you interact and respond to the actor's behaviour during the consultation. You are usually not required to examine a patient and little marks will be given for the clinical diagnosis or management. You should all be familiar with simulated patients, as actors are often used to play patients in medical OSCE exams. The actors are highly trained and will express a wide range of emotions just as a real patient would. If you approach the task with the right mind-set, it is usually easy to imagine them as a real-life patient. Your aim is to respond to the simulated patient appropriately, as a doctor would in a real-life consultation. Hopefully, this is a role that you are all very familiar with and should not have any difficultly fulfilling. There are however, some distinct differences between a hospital-based consultation and a general practice consultation, which we will go on to discuss later. To help you make the most of the exercises in this chapter you can download blank mark schemes from www.bpp.com/freehealthresources

What do the simulated exercises involve?

The simulated exercises may involve a consultation with a patient, a patient's family member or perhaps a work colleague. The role of the patient/relative/colleague is usually played by a trained actor (the simulator). However, it is also possible to have this role played by an assessor, although this is not common. In the room, you will also have one or two trained assessors with you. These assessors are usually doctors such as General Practitioners or Consultants with specific training for this purpose. However, they can also be trained educational psychologists. The assessors will make sure you understand the instructions; however they will remain silent throughout the exercise and will not be involved in the role play.

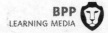

The 'patient' has been given a defined role to play which will usually bring out specific issues. They are given instructions on not only what to say, but also how they should look and what demeanour they should express. They are also occasionally told to withhold certain information unless you ask them the correct question or make them feel comfortable enough to tell you. The simulator will also make an assessment of your performance commenting especially on how you made them feel during the exercise, for example, if you made them feel comfortable, if they felt you were genuinely concerned and interested in what they had to say. These comments may, but not always, be used when assessing your competencies.

Format of the simulated exercises

The precise format of your three patient simulated exercises will vary across deaneries. You will be given a brief; a sheet of paper or card with the background to the case written on it. This will normally be a short paragraph, however it may even be a simple sentence such as 'Mr Smith, aged 46 has come to see you with regards to his chest pain.' For most of the deaneries you will be given five minutes before the exercise starts to read the brief and information given to you. These five minutes are crucially important and we will explain later how to gain as much information as you can from the brief and use this time to your advantage.

You will also have an opportunity during your five minutes to re-arrange the furniture in the room if required. The importance of this will be discussed in more detail later. The assessors will ensure that you have understood the information given to you and you will have a chance to ask them any questions if something in the brief is not clear before you start. The patient or simulator at this time is usually outside the room and after reading the brief you will be expected to invite the patient into the room.

The actual time allocated to the consultation may vary between deaneries. For most, there will be 20 minutes to complete the consultation but you do not have to use all of the time available. Some deaneries use an OSCE-like format where you will have ten minutes to complete the consultation. Therefore, it is important to find out in advance from your deanery how much time you will have for the exercise.

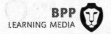

You will be expected to bring the consultation to a natural close yourself within your allocated time. The assessors may give you a warning when your time is about to run out or they may simply not say anything until your time is up. If you are in the OSCE-type exam a bell may simply ring at the end of the allocated time. To avoid being caught out and having your consultation ended abruptly by the assessors, it is a good idea to keep an eye on the time yourself. Therefore, you may want to bring a digital watch or stop clock with you. Failing this you could ask the assessors to give you a warning when you have a certain amount of time remaining.

Common topics in the simulated exercises

In general, there are two types of exercise that you may encounter in the assessment. The first is that of a normal consultation where the patient comes to you with a particular presenting complaint and you are expected to come to a diagnosis and management plan. Although the presenting complaint may be a medical one, there are usually hidden psychosocial issues or an underlying patient concern that you need to elicit and address. As the exercise is designed to assess your communication skills and how you interact with patients, you are unlikely to encounter a case with a complicated medical history where the diagnosis is unclear. This is simply because that type of case would be assessing your medical knowledge and clinical skills which has already been tested in the previous stages of the assessment. Therefore, the presenting complaint is usually a simple and common problem encountered frequently in general practice; such as a headache or being tired all the time. Once again you will not be marked on the medical aspect of your diagnosis or management plan and the focus is more on your ability to establish a rapport with the patient and elicit their worries and concerns.

The second type of exercise you may encounter is one where you are expected to explain a diagnosis or a test result to a patient. This is likely to be a common diagnosis in general practice, for example explaining to a patient that they are asthmatic, but may also involve breaking bad news. These types of cases give you a better opportunity to demonstrate your empathy and communication skills and are common in the patient simulated exercise.

 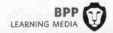

In theory any case encountered in general practice may come up. However, some common cases are:

- Having to explain a condition (usually chronic) to a patient
- Breaking bad news
- Dealing with an error or a mistake made by either yourself or another doctor
- Dealing with a complaint
- Dealing with a difficult, angry or demanding patient
- Explaining a test result or procedure
- Dealing with a patient who has poor compliance with a treatment, e.g. does not use their inhalers appropriately
- Dealing with psychosocial issues

Assessment criteria for the simulated exercise

As stated in the introduction of this book, the National Person Specification is used to assess the whole of the Stage 3 application process. The two different parts of the assessment will test different criteria within this person specification; however there will be some overlap. In general, the simulated exercise is primarily designed to assess:

Empathy and sensitivity

- Having a caring manner as a whole
- Understanding and appreciating the patient's/relative's/colleague's concerns and the ability to reassure them
- Understanding the effect the patient's symptoms or concerns are having on the physical, emotional and social aspects of their life
- Involving the patient in management decisions taking into account their personal beliefs and wishes
- Establishing a rapport with the patient/relative/colleague
- Remaining attentive to the patient/relative/colleague throughout the consultation
- Using the correct body language and non-verbal gestures to put the patient/relative/colleague at ease and offer support or reassurance at the appropriate times.

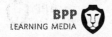

Communication skills

- Explaining things clearly and not in medical jargon
- Using silence appropriately and showing that you are listening to the patient
- Using non-verbal behaviour such as body language to aid effective communication
- Using supportive words and open-ended questions to encourage and aid dialogue
- Adapting your language and manner to the situation
- Ensuring that the patient has understood what has been said

Coping with pressure

- Keeping calm throughout the consultation
- Dealing with a variety of patient emotions appropriately, including anger
- Dealing with difficult patient presentations and eliciting the patient's beliefs and concerns in these scenarios
- Being flexible when challenged
- Maintaining your perspective when under pressure

Professional integrity

- Acting within your professional boundaries and realising when you are out of your depth
- Demonstrating respect for the patient taking into account their feelings and wishes
- Acknowledging your own errors and taking responsibility for them
- Showing confidence in your own judgement and decisions
- Being accepting of others
- Making adequate arrangements should the worst happen (safety-netting) and arranging appropriate follow up where necessary

Organisation and planning

- Finishing the consultation smoothly within the time allocated

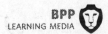

Clinical knowledge and expertise
- Coming to a correct diagnosis and form an appropriate management plan

For most of the scenarios you will be assessed on the first four criteria only:
- Empathy and sensitivity
- Communication Skills
- Coping with Pressure
- Professional Integrity

However, the simulated exercises you are given will differ and therefore will assess these competencies to different degrees, depending on the scenario. For example, if you have to admit that a mistake has been made to a patient, this will primarily assess your professional integrity and how you cope under pressure. However, it will also obviously address your communications skills as this may be a sensitive subject and you will need to show empathy towards the situation. A scenario where you need to break bad news to a patient on the other hand, will concentrate primarily on your empathy and communication skills, assessing your professional integrity and your ability to cope under pressure to a lesser degree.

Although you will score points for finishing the consultation within the allocated time and coming to a suitable diagnosis and management plan, little marks will be given for this. You may have also noticed that problem-solving, managing others and learning/professional development are not mentioned above. This is because these aspects are usually tested more formally in the prioritisation exercises, which are more suitable to assess these criteria. However, you may encounter a simulated exercise that addresses these, although it is unlikely to be in any detail.

Mark scheme for the simulated exercises

Many candidates naturally would like to know what the mark scheme is for the simulated exercise. Unfortunately, there is no set mark scheme and the criteria they are assessing will vary from case to case as previously explained. You may be assessed on all four of the person specifications listed above or perhaps on only two or

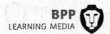

three of them. The likelihood however is that you will be given a case that can address all four competencies: empathy/sensitivity, communication skills, professional integrity and coping under pressure, as these criteria can easily be tested by the simulated exercise.

For each person specification there are between 6–8 different points that were considered appropriate examples of demonstrating that particular competency. Similarly, in the assessment there will be several opportunities in the exercise to exhibit particular criteria of the person specification, and you will be expected to show this skill at all of these opportunities. For example, if the assessors were assessing your communication skills for example, you would not be marked as fulfilling the criteria if you managed to explain things in non-medical terms, but did not listen to the patient or make sure that they understood what you had said. Therefore, you need to be consistent in demonstrating that you are competent in a particular skill.

The exact description of what the assessors are looking for within each person specification and the number of points that you need to address will depend on the actual case. From previous mark schemes however, the assessors have assessed about six different points for each of the various person specifications. This means that for each of the specifications: empathy/sensitivity, communication skills, coping under pressure and professional integrity, there will be six different points that you need to exhibit to show the assessors that you have achieved that competency. For each of the points you can be marked as follows:

1. **Showing a clear strength in demonstrating the skill**
   This is the highest mark obtainable and shows that you have shown the assessors throughout the exercise that you are highly competent in this skill.

2. **Showing a mixed demonstration of the skill**
   This means that you have exhibited some evidence of having the necessary skill at certain points of the consultation, but it is not consistent enough to be marked as a clear strength. This may be because you have excelled in some parts of the consultation but not in others.

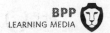

3. **Showing a need for development of the skill**
   This means that you have made some attempt to demonstrate the competency assessed. However you have not proved at any point that you are competent enough in the skill for it to be considered a strength and it is clear that you need further development.

4. **Showing no evidence of the skill**
   This is the lowest grade and is given when you have not showed any evidence of the skill at all.

Some deaneries use a modification of this scheme and instead use these rankings. They are essentially the same as the ones just discussed:

1. Very good demonstration of competence suggesting a strength
2. Sufficient demonstration of competence
3. Insufficient demonstration of competence
4. No evidence of competence

For clarity, a hypothetical example of a possible mark scheme which assesses empathy and sensitivity is shown below. This mark scheme would be similar for each of the other person specifications addressed.

Empathy and sensitivity mark scheme

		No evidence	Development Need	Mixed Demonstration	Strength
a	Generated a safe and trusting atmosphere				
b	Acted in a caring and non-judgemental manner				
c	Responded to the patient's concerns with interest and understanding				
d	Established a rapport with the patient				
e	Co-operated with the patient taking their beliefs and wishes into consideration				
f	Reassured the patient				

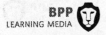

Obviously if you clearly score 'strength' for each of the points, you will pass the simulated exercise. However remember that each of the person specifications may be tested in each of the three exercises and that your overall scores on the day are triangulated. This means that you can still be selected overall, even if you have not scored 'strength' for each of the points within the consultation exercise, as you may have scored highly in the two other exercises. Unfortunately, you do need to score above a minimum level in each exercise to be selected for training. This 'minimum level' will vary across Deaneries. Your score will also be ranked against the other candidates, and the score needed to pass will depend on the quality of the candidates present. Therefore, it is best to go into the exercise aiming to meet all of the necessary criteria, but not being too disheartened if a certain part of the consultation does not go as well.

There are various different ways to approach the simulated exercise and a very structured approach is provided later that will help to ensure that you score all the points required to be successful. The suggested approach may seem very detailed; however it is impossible to ascertain which case you will face on the day and therefore exactly what the assessors will be marking you on. Therefore, by providing you with a very detailed approach that can be applied to any scenario to the consultation, you will be able to prepare yourself for any eventuality.

However, to begin with, it is useful to discuss how the consultation in the simulated exercise will differ from the usual consultations you are used to within hospital medicine. This may highlight bad habits that you will need to change for the assessment. It is also useful to be aware of the basic principles of the communication skills that will be fundamental for passing the simulated exercise.

General practice consultations versus hospital based clerkings

There are distinct differences between the way a general practitioner and a hospital doctor consult. Most of you, as hospital doctors, are familiar with dealing with patients referred by their GP and are adept at taking medical histories from these patients. By the time the patient is referred to you, the GP has usually made

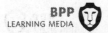

some sort of diagnosis or differential diagnosis and you have all the resources available to you to investigate the problem further. Your job is basically to see whether you agree or disagree with the diagnosis by taking a very problem-based history. There is little emphasis on how the patient feels or what they feel is wrong with them and most of your history involves asking the patient questions where they simply answer yes or no. Once the diagnosis is clear, a management decision is made and the patient is rarely ever involved in making decisions on their management or asked how they feel about the various options. This approach to the consultation is very doctor-centred. By this we mean that the consultation involves the doctor being seen as the expert and the patient is simply expected to co-operate with the decision made. The whole point of the consultation in these circumstances is to come to some sort of organic diagnosis.

General practice is not the same. Patients often present to primary care with very vague symptoms and as a GP you need to be able to use your communication skills to explore this further. Patients often present with psychosomatic illness which can be very challenging. Although those of you who have worked in hospital medicine may be familiar with the patient who is convinced there is something wrong with them despite their tests being negative; your job was simply to exclude any medical illness. Therefore, you could simply discharge them after you had excluded any physical problem suggesting that they follow up with their GP. However, you are now their GP and need to know how to deal with these patients. You need to learn how to ask the right questions; trying to understand the reasons behind their presentation and addressing the issues and beliefs that are behind their physical symptoms.

It is also important in general practice to involve the patient in the management decisions as opposed to dictating to the patient what you feel is best. This usually involves giving the patient different choices in how they could be managed and asking them which option they would like to try. This sort of approach to the consultation is more patient-centred: that is, it encourages the patient to voice their own feelings and concerns and allows them to have some sort of control over the outcome of the consultation.

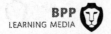

Although patient-centred consultations and communication skills may be something that you have little experience in as a hospital doctor, it is something that can be easily learned. There are a wide range of techniques you can use to improve your communication skills that are discussed in this chapter. However, the key to implementing these skills is to practise. These skills cannot be learnt from a book or lecture. You can learn the basics but you need to put the theory into action. However, before you go on to practise your skills in the role play exercises lets address the basics.

Concepts for the simulated exercises
Safety-netting

Unlike hospital-based medicine, general practice often involves making diagnoses and management plans with little access to immediate investigations such as blood tests or X-rays. It is very important to ensure that you 'safety-net'. This is preparing for the unexpected in case anything goes wrong. This may be that the patient's condition worsens or that the patient starts to exhibit other symptoms that may be indicative of another condition. Therefore, at the end of the consultation it is particularly important to ensure that you have given the patient the specific circumstances under which they need to come back and the time frame for this. An example of safety-netting may be telling a patient with a cough who you have diagnosed with a chest infection:

> *'Mr Smith, should you develop any shortness of breath, cough up any blood or develop a high fever I would like you to see a doctor immediately. Also should you not feel any better after the seven day course of antibiotics I would also like you to come back to see me.'*

Safety-netting will be discussed in more detail later.

Ideas, concerns and expectations

These are very important concepts in general practice and ones you may not be familiar with as a hospital doctor. The concept of the patient-centred consultation has already been mentioned. This involves treating the patient as a whole and taking into account their beliefs, thoughts and feelings during the consultation.

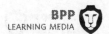

Having done so, you can tailor the consultation to incorporate the patient's beliefs and can take their feelings into consideration when formulating management decisions. You therefore need to identify these thoughts and feelings so that this process is possible. This can be achieved by asking the patient about their ideas, concerns and expectations (ICE). This can be described as follows:

Ideas: This involves the patient's beliefs about what they think is wrong with them or even why they think it is happening to them. For example, a patient with back pain may feel they have a slipped disc because someone at work had something similar or because they read about it online.

Questions you can ask to decipher the patient's ideas about their symptoms may be:

> - *'Sometimes people have thoughts on what can be causing their symptoms; have you any thoughts on what could be causing yours?'*
> - *'Have you had any thoughts on what you think might be happening?'*

Concerns: This is what the patient is worried about, e.g. what condition their symptoms may represent or what may happen as a result of their condition. It may be similar to the belief or it may be different. For example, a smoker with a cough may believe they have a chest infection but may secretly be worried that they have cancer.

Questions you can ask to determine what the patient may be concerned about are:

> - *'Was there any particular condition you were worried this may be?'*
> - *'Have you had any concerns as to what this may be or what may happen?'*

Expectations: This is what the patient is expecting to happen as a result of the consultation, e.g. a referral, an X-ray or blood test or perhaps a prescription for something. Patients often have

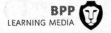

preconceived ideas not only as to what is wrong with them, but also as to what they want to happen. For example, a lot of patients who have simple coughs and colds may have already formed the expectation that they should receive antibiotics.

Questions that are useful to identify the patient's expectations are:

> - *'Have you had any thoughts on how we should proceed with this matter?'*
> - *'Have you had any thoughts on how you feel I can help you with this problem?'*

These questions are extremely important, as unless you can identify the patient's ideas, concerns and expectations you cannot ensure that you have reassured them adequately. For example, a patient with a simple upper respiratory tract infection may come to see you. That same patient may believe that they have a chest infection. They are worried about this because they have had a chest infection before and did not see a doctor resulting in them being admitted to hospital with pneumonia. In addition, their father has recently died of lung cancer and as they are a smoker they are secretly worried it may be cancer. Therefore, they are expecting to have an X-ray to exclude cancer as well as a course of antibiotics for their chest infection.

You on the other hand, having not elicited any of this, have simply examined them and found that their chest was clear. As a result you have told them they have a viral illness and that no further action is needed. Although medically speaking you have identified the illness and provided an appropriate management plan, the patient is likely to have left unsatisfied. This is because you have not explained to the patient that they have a simple upper respiratory tract infection, taking into account their belief that it is a chest infection and possibly cancer. Therefore, you needed to have explained to the patient what an upper respiratory tract infection was, why it did not require antibiotics or an X-ray, and why you are certain they do not have cancer or a chest infection for them to have been reassured. This is distinctively different to just telling them 'you have a virus, go home and rest' and illustrates why

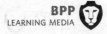

asking the necessary questions is fundamental to fully addressing the patient's concerns.

Hidden agenda

The hidden agenda is closely linked to the concept of ideas, concerns and expectations and comes up frequently in the simulated assessment. However, unlike a simple belief or concern it is more difficult to elicit and is often not revealed by the patient unless they feel comfortable enough to tell you. The hidden agenda is essentially the real reason as to why the patient is coming to see you. However, it is not the patient's 'presenting complaint' and you have to use your communication skills to first, figure out that there may be a hidden agenda, and second, to try and identify what the agenda is.

An example of a hidden agenda may be a patient who comes to you presenting with menstrual problems, however is secretly being abused by her partner. If you simply take what she says on face value you will never identify the real reason as to why she has come to see you. You will need to pick up on both verbal and non-verbal clues that something else is going on. For example, she may seem very nervous which is unusual if she is simply coming to discuss her periods or she may seem very depressed. The actors in the simulation exercise are very convincing and they will exhibit signs of anger, nervousness and depression just as patients would do in real life. It is important to identify this from the beginning and to comment on it to gain more information, e.g. 'you seem very upset today'. This will show the patient that you recognise and are in touch with how they are feeling and will encourage them to open up more.

To reveal a hidden agenda you also need to make sure you establish a good psychosocial history to see if there are any other problems. This is distinctly different to the social history you take in your medical clerking when you may ask who they live with, if they smoke or if they have any pets. It involves assessing how the presenting complaint may be affecting their lives emotionally, financially, psychologically and spiritually. For example, it may be the question, 'how is this affecting your relationship with your partner?' that reveals the abuse the patient is suffering.

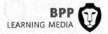

It is also important to make the patient feel comfortable as the actors in the assessment are often told that they will only reveal certain information if the candidate makes them feel comfortable to do so. Thus you will need to use certain skills within the consultation to put the patient, relative or colleague at ease in order to tease out this sensitive information. Therefore, as you can see, the consultation in the simulated exercise is not a simple medical history and usually always involves some sort of hidden agenda or psychosocial issue.

We will now go on to discuss the skills needed in order to identify these issues and pass the simulated exercise.

Skills required for the consultation
Active listening

Listening is one of the most important skills in general practice. However, in everyday life people rarely listen attentively to each other, e.g. they may be thinking of other things or wondering what to say next. Therefore part of being able to effectively communicate is not just your ability to listen but to *actively* listen. This is a more structured approach to listening where you not only use silence, but also really try to understand what the speaker is saying and how they are feeling. This may involve picking up on verbal and non verbal clues while the other person is talking, but also 'reflecting back' (see later) what the person has said to show understanding. Active listening is important as it avoids misunderstanding, but also shows that you are really in tune with the other person's concerns, which encourages the person to open up more. Therefore, it is a fundamental skill in general practice which allows you to connect with the patient and develop a rapport with them. In doing so, you can establish the real reasons behind the patient's presentation and are more likely to be able to address the patient's concerns.

During the simulated exercise the assessors will be assessing your communication skills and not your ability to take a medical history. Therefore, it is likely that as the actor speaks they will be giving you clues about their underlying issues or concerns. If you interrupt continuously or do not pay attention, you are likely to miss out on these clues. You need to keep an open mind and actively listen

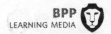

and look out for clues that will help you identify what is really going on. Do not let yourself get distracted.

Also remember that there may be certain issues that are difficult to discuss, e.g. domestic violence or sexual issues. If you interrupt at the wrong moment it could be the difference between them telling you the real reason for their presentation and them walking out of the room or pretending there is something else wrong. Therefore, try to be silent initially when the patient is talking. Do not rush to take your usual 'medical history' but let them talk and gain as much information as you can. Try not to interrupt until their conversation has come to a natural end. This is actually a lot harder than it seems, and as most of you as busy hospital doctors, will be used to rushing to take a history, it may take a bit of practice. This is something you can work on in small groups, but it is also something you can try with your own hospital patients if time permits.

As we stated previously, active listening requires silence but also observing body language and behaviour, ie looking out for verbal and non-verbal clues. For example, does the actor seem like they are hiding something, e.g. by avoiding eye contact? This may give you a clue that perhaps there may be a hidden agenda. Do they seem nervous? Perhaps this may mean that they are worried that there is something seriously wrong with them or that it is an embarrassing or sensitive issue. Have they already diagnosed themselves, e.g. 'doctor I have a chest infection.' Why do they think that? Have they had a chest infection before? What was their experience when that happened, e.g. did they end up very unwell and therefore are naturally anxious to prevent this from happening again? Do they keep repeating themselves? Is this because they feel they are not being listened to or is this because they are trying to tell us something? Everything the patient, relative or colleague says or doesn't say is important. This is because it will help you to understand where they are coming from, and will also allow you to tailor the consultation to take into account how they are thinking and feeling.

Active listening also involves showing that you are interested in what they have to say and that you understand what they are trying to tell you. Therefore, be aware of your own body language when

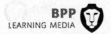

listening. Lean forward to show you are being attentive and try to maintain eye contact to show you are interested. It is easy to drift off or lose concentration when the patient is talking for a while especially when you are nervous. In certain circumstances it may be appropriate to nod your head to show you are acknowledging and understanding what they have said. At other times it may be appropriate to use simple phrases like 'hmm' or an 'oh dear' once again to show you have heard what they have said and are acknowledging how they must feel.

Open-ended questions

How you phrase a question will determine the quantity and the quality of the information you receive. Medical clerkings are designed to gain specific diagnostic information and therefore involves a great deal of closed questions, e.g. do you have chest pain? Do you have a fever? These 'closed questions' can really only be answered with a 'yes' or 'no' and therefore do not allow you to obtain any extra information. However, with the simulated exercise as with general practice consultations, it is important to hear the story. You want to know how the patient, relative or colleague is feeling and what is worrying them as well as trying to figure out the diagnosis. Open-ended questions are useful for this purpose as they are less specific in what they are asking for and allow a more detailed answer. This may give you extra valuable information. An example of an open-ended question that is in direct contrast to the closed question asked about chest pain would be:

> *'Can you tell me more about your chest pain?'*

Open-ended questions are very important when asking the patient, relative or colleague the reason for them coming to see you. For example, you may be given a brief in the assessment that states that a patient has come to you today for a repeat prescription. However, the actor's instructions are that there is really another issue that they want to discuss but will only do so if you ask them the correct questions. Using an open-ended question such as, 'can you tell me what has brought you here today?', allows them to tell their story and mention if they have any other issue. Their response may also give you a clue that there is something else going on. However, if you ask a closed question such as, 'have you

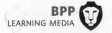

come for your repeat prescription today?', you may have simply been answered with a 'yes'. Therefore although there was really a hidden agenda as to why they were attending today, you have not given them the opportunity to express themselves and have therefore missed the point completely.

It is also useful to ask open-ended questions after your opening statement to encourage the patient to tell you more. You can often do this if a patient seems to close up or perhaps does not reveal much initially. Sometimes a patient may spend a long time going into detail about what is bothering them after a simple prompt of 'how can I help you today?' However, occasionally a patient may initially reveal very little information to the same question, such as 'it's my cough doctor.' Here the use of an open-ended question, such as 'can you tell me more about your cough?', may encourage the patient to tell you their concerns and what they feel the cough represents. Obviously if you go straight into closed questions such as 'are you short of breath?' or 'do you smoke?' you will miss hearing what the patient is thinking and feeling and will not address the necessary issues.

Obviously there are times where it is appropriate to use closed questions especially when you are trying to exclude any serious 'red-flag symptoms.' It would be appropriate in this same scenario to ask a patient with a cough, 'have you coughed up any blood?'. However, you should try to leave these questions until later on in the consultation, once you have spent some time listening to the patient and encouraging them to tell you their story. This will become muchclearer later when we discuss how to structure your consultations.

Clarifying/reflecting back

This is another useful tool which forms part of your active listening and not only avoids misunderstandings but shows that you have really listened and have understood. This in itself can often make the patient sufficiently comfortable to reveal sensitive information to you.

Therefore, it is useful after the patient has told you their story to just summarise or clarify what they have said. This can be particularly useful in the assessment when you are nervous and

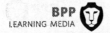

may have misheard or not completely understood what the patient has said. An example of this may be:

> 'So Mr Smith, just so that I can make sure that I have understood you correctly, you have had diarrhoea for one week now since your return from a trip to Kenya and are naturally very concerned that you may have picked up an infection out there.'

By doing this you have showed the patient you have listened to what they have said, and are also giving them an opportunity to correct any misunderstandings before you go on to make a formal diagnosis and explain the management to them.

The skill of 'reflecting back' is similar, however here you simply repeat the last sentence or phrase followed by a pause. This can often be used to gain more information without the need to ask a specific question and shows you have picked up on their comment. This is because the patient, relative or colleague usually fills the pause with either an explanation or an extension of what they were saying. For example, a patient with a headache may simply say to you, 'I'm worried doctor'. By reflecting back this statement to the patient by saying, 'you said you were worried (pause)', the patient may say 'yes doctor I'm worried I have a tumour' and go on to tell you why. Thus, you have gained the information without necessarily asking the patient what they are worried about. This does not mean it would be wrong to ask the patient what they are concerned about, it is just another way of obtaining the necessary information from them.

Empathy

It is essential to be empathic during the simulated exercise and you will be marked on this. It may be tested in something obvious such as breaking bad news to a patient, or it may be a more subtle situation such as a single mother with a cold who secretly is struggling to cope. You can show empathy in several ways both verbally and non-verbally. It may be by a gentle hand on a patient's shoulder who is upset or an empathic comment such as, 'I can understand that must be terribly hard for you'. Always remember to put yourself in the patient's shoes and to try and

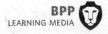

understand the impact their symptoms or complaint is having on their quality of life.

Summarising

Summarising is a useful tool within the consultation that will show both the assessor and the patient, relative or colleague that you have understood each other. It is very similar to clarifying in that you repeat (summarise) what has been said to ensure that you have understood what they have come to see about and what their concerns are. However, unlike clarifying, which shows that *you* have actively listened and understood what that *they* have said, summarising can be used to ensure that the patient, relative or colleague has understood *you*.

This is particularly important at the end of the consultation as you need to ensure that everything you have said has been understood correctly. Thus, you may need to ask the actor if they would be able to summarise what has been said today just to make sure that you have both understood each other correctly. This is an excellent way to prove to the assessor that you have communicated effectively and that the patient, relative or colleague understands and is happy with the management plan.

General tips for the simulated exercises
Be yourself

The simulated exercise is designed to try to recreate a typical consultation within a general practice setting. It is important to try and be as natural as possible and to try and act exactly as you would in a consultation. Although a very structured approach to the simulated exercise will be discussed, you are an individual and will have your unique personal traits that can be incorporated into the consultation. Therefore, if you have your own way of explaining things that you feel comfortable with then do so. This may be through the use of analogies, e.g. likening white cells in the blood to 'soldiers' fighting against infection or perhaps diagrams. Some of you may write down certain advice while others may prefer giving out leaflets. The main point is that you should try to explain conditions and management decisions in ways that can be understood.

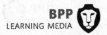

The simulated patients, relatives or colleagues

It is easy to become distracted on the day due to nerves. It is also difficult for some people to imagine an actor as a real life patient, relative or colleague, and as such you may miss out on certain clues or perhaps feel uncomfortable doing things that usually come naturally, e.g. handing a tissue to an upset patient. The actors however, are usually very convincing and will express a wide range of emotions for you to pick up on. It is important to treat them like real 'people' and not to change your behaviour because they are an 'actor'. Be prepared for the actors to express themselves in ways your patients, their relatives or your colleagues would. Consequently, they may burst into tears or become angry and start shouting at you. This can easily distract you from your train of thought if you are not prepared for it. For some of you however, the assessors may take on the acting role and this will make 'being yourself' even harder. Try not to become distracted by this and imagine that you are in your normal day at work acting accordingly.

Improvise

Although the exercise is designed to 'simulate' a typical consultation there may be certain tools you normally use in your consultation that are not at your disposal. For example, you are unlikely to have all your equipment with you on the day and are also unlikely to have books such as the British National Formulary (BNF) or patient leaflets. Therefore if you need to look something up in the BNF as you are unsure of a side effect or dosage of a medication, then you may wish to improvise and tell the patient that you will find this information out after your discussion. If you normally use patient leaflets in your consultation you can also improvise by saying, 'before you leave I will give you a leaflet on your condition.' The point is you need to be as natural as possible and it is a lot easier if you just follow your own consultation style. Therefore do not get distracted if you are asked something you do not know the answer to, or if you do not have something at your disposal that ideally you would like to have, e.g. a placebo inhaler when explaining asthma to a patient. It is perfectly acceptable to tell the patient that you will get this information or tool for them at a later time.

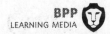

Also, despite the fact that little marks are given for the clinical diagnosis during the patient simulated exercise, there may be times where you would wish to examine a patient, as you would in your every day consultations. Although you would be very unlikely to get a case where you need to examine a patient, it may be appropriate to mention that you would like to examine them for completeness sake. For example, you may have a case where you need to break bad news to a patient that he has lung cancer. However, if he tells you that he is still very short of breath it may be appropriate to suggest that you will examine his chest after the consultation. This is likely to be what you would do in reality to ensure that he does not have any serious breathing difficulty or perhaps a superimposed chest infection. It is completely appropriate to improvise on these occasions, and mention to the patient after you have ensured that he has understood his diagnosis and management, that you will examine his chest in another room. Under no circumstances however should you attempt to undress the actor to examine him or her in the assessment.

Perform on the day

On the day you do need to make sure that you clearly exhibit all the necessary skills to the assessors. You may remember having to do this during the clinical OSCEs you sat during medical school. In these exams you had to examine the patient in a very structured and organised way to clearly show the assessor that you were competent in that clinical skill. Some of you may remember that when examining the abdomen you had to kneel on the floor and had to examine with your right hand to pass that station. As a result, simply coming to the correct diagnosis was not sufficient to pass the station alone. Your whole method of examining the patient and the comments used were important, and everything you did that led up to that diagnosis had to be done in the correct way. Therefore, the mark sheet was a series of boxes, with a box ticked every time you correctly performed a part of the assessment or correctly commented on a clinical sign. To pass the station overall you needed to have a certain number of boxes ticked, and it was your overall performance that was important.

The simulated exercise is very similar in this respect. However, unlike a multiple choice question exam where there is only a 'yes' or 'no' answer, the marking of this exam is quite subjective. By this

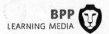

we mean that it is really up to the assessor's discretion to determine whether you have met the specific criteria or not. This means that you need to clearly show theassessors that you are competent in that area. If you remember the mark scheme discussed, it is quite easy to partially demonstrate a competency and miss out on being assessed as having a clear strength. Therefore, to ensure that there is no question about your competency, you will often have to say or do very specific tasks to ensure that you have met the requirement.

For example, there may be a particular case that is assessing your communication skills and you ensure that a patient has understood the information you have given to them. To illustrate clearly that you have met this requirement you may need to ask the patient to summarise what you have said, e.g. 'just to ensure that we are both clear on what has been said would you like to summarise what we have discussed today?' Hopefully, the patient will then reiterate correctly what you have said, demonstrating that they have understood everything clearly, and you will be scored as having a clear strength in this skill. This is distinctively different from simply asking the patient, 'do you understand?' Here the patient may answer 'yes' even if they haven't fully understood. This would not truly prove to the assessor that you have communicated the information effectively and that the patient understands. As a result, you may only be marked as having a mixed demonstration of the skill or even a developmental need. Therefore, you will need to make sure that you take active steps to demonstrate each of the competencies fully.

Read the brief carefully

The brief is designed to give you a short introduction to what your case involves. It usually consists of only a few sentences or a short paragraph giving you the background to the case. The actors however are usually given a very long and detailed brief informing them on what to do and to say and under what circumstances they will reveal certain information to you. Hence the case is rarely ever as simple as what you have been told in the brief.

Although you do not want to assume what the case involves before you see the patient, it is useful to have an idea of what could potentially be asked of you. If you have some possible ideas of

 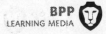

what the case involves or what the deeper issue may be, you can prepare yourself mentally for what clues may be relevant from the patient or what questions you need to ask. Always bear in mind that you are unlikely to be faced with a case which simply involves making a clinical diagnosis; there is usually an underlying psychosocial issue or something slightly more complicated going on. Also always remember that the information provided in the brief is always correct. Therefore if you are told that a result is normal or that the patient does not have a certain symptom, this is the case. Do not waste precious time asking again for information that you have been already given.

Example Brief 1

Doctor's brief

> Mrs Smith, aged 27, has come to see you with regards to an occasional dry cough she has had since her return from Kenya two weeks ago. She had been seen previously by one of your colleagues who reassured her that her chest X-ray and spirometry were all normal. She remains well within herself and has no temperatures, haemoptysis or shortness of breath. She has never smoked.

The way to approach reading the brief is to read it in its entirety once and then read it again highlighting the salient points. The easiest way to do this is to underline key words or sentences and make notes as to what you feel could be important. Remember that even basic details such as the name may be important, especially if it gives you a clue to the ethnicity of the patient, as this may help you understand some of their health beliefs.

In this particular scenario the following information could perhaps have some relevance:

Mrs Smith, aged 27

Medically speaking her young age would make a diagnosis of lung cancer unlikely. As she is young and from her title you know that she is married perhaps you need to explore the psychosocial impact of this cough on her life, e.g. does she have young children and is she finding it hard to cope? Is she having marital difficulty?

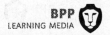

Occasional dry cough

As the cough is dry we can already exclude certain conditions where we would expect a productive cough, e.g. a chest infection. However, as the cough is only occasional, why is the patient so worried about it? Perhaps she is concerned about a particular diagnosis or perhaps it is affecting her quality of life? You may need to find this out later.

Returned from Kenya two weeks ago

Medically speaking this may be of relevance; however we must remember that this case is unlikely to simply involve making a clinical diagnosis. Perhaps the patient is worried that she has caught a serious infection as she has been abroad? Has her concern been identified and addressed if this is the case?

She has been seen previously by one of your colleagues

The fact that she is coming back to see you when your colleague has been dealing with the matter tells you that something is wrong. It may be that she simply could not arrange an appointment to see your colleague or it may be that she was not satisfied with your colleague's advice. This may be because your colleague did not explain the cause of the cough properly or perhaps did not address the patient's concerns. It may even be that she had a hidden agenda that was not elicited by your colleague. It would therefore be sensible to ask her what she has been told by your colleague and what she understood by this discussion, to help you identify why she is still not satisfied by the advice she has been given.

A chest X-ray and spirometry were all normal

This is telling you that you have excluded any serious medical condition such as asthma, malignancy or infection. Therefore it would be inappropriate to take a long medical history from this patient and you should trust that information in the brief is correct. As it seems that there is not going to be an obvious medical cause for this cough, it indicates that there may be more of a psychosocial issue. Therefore you may need to delve a little deeper into what is concerning the patient and how this cough is affecting her.

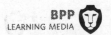

She remains well and has no temperatures, haemoptysis or shortness of breath. She has never smoked

This again rules out most serious conditions and is telling us that her symptoms have not changed. This information is being given to you for a reason and as stated before is accurate. Therefore, there is no need to take a long medical history and ask about any red flag symptoms as we are already told that there aren't any.

It is now possible to summarise the information gained from reading the brief. You are presented with a young patient who has recently come back from holiday who is experiencing an occasional dry cough. Her investigations are normal and you have excluded any serious medical condition. She has already been seen by another colleague and reassured that her test results were normal; however there is definitely an issue that has not been addressed as she has come to see you with the same problem. Although you are unaware of the exact issue at this moment; her age, marital status and her recent trip to Kenya may be of some relevance. You should be prepared to ask her how this cough may be affecting her home and personal life and if there is anything that she may be worried about. It should also make you more aware of any clues she may give you which could include that she is having difficulties coping with her cough or that she is concerned about something, such as her recent trip abroad.

Although this may not be the exact issue at hand, thinking about what possible issues may be relevant can make you more alert to certain clues that could tell you what really is going on. Therefore reading the brief carefully can be more useful than you think.

Keep to time

Bringing the consultation to its natural end within the allocated time is not easy and involves a lot of practice. The aim is to ask all of the relevant questions and be able to finish the consultation smoothly within the time you are given. However, if you are running slightly behind it looks more professional to realise this and bring the consultation to a close naturally, than to be stopped mid-sentence by the assessors as your time is up. Therefore, when you practise your role play scenarios you will need to do this under timed conditions, so that you get into the habit of being able to

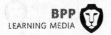

consult within the short-time frame. Candidates commonly spend a lot of time taking long drawn out medical histories and leave little time to explore the patient's concerns or the psychosocial aspect of the case. Consequently, try to get into the habit of asking a few relevant medical questions in your history that may help you come to a diagnosis, as opposed to taking the full medical clerking types of history that you are used to.

For example, if a mother brings her child to you with a chronic cough you are likely to want to exclude infection or perhaps asthma. Ask about fevers, shortness of breath, wheeze and any family history of asthma. It is not necessary to start asking about sputum colour or start doing a systems review for every possible symptom. Similarly, if you have an elderly man who has no other relevant past medical history with a chronic cough you are likely to want to rule out malignancy. Hence you will need to ask about smoking, weight loss and haemoptysis to exclude this. It is not necessary to ask about whether he has any pets at home; whether he is suffering from paroxysmal nocturnal dyspnoea; whether he has palpitations or perform a full cardiovascular systems review. This is not to say that those symptoms are not important; but you need to be able to focus your history to exclude what are the most possible likely diagnoses in that particular case.

It is also useful to bring a small clock or watch on the day to remind you to keep to time. Initially when the patient is telling you their story, do not look at the watch continuously, as you will lose marks for breaking eye contact and poor body language. However, it is very useful towards the end of the consultation when you tend to take control of the consultation and do most of the talking. If your deanery allows you 20 minutes for the exercise, it is advisable in the last five minutes to begin asking the patient to summarise the consultation and ensure that they have understood what you have said. If you are in the ten minute style OSCE you may wish to initiate this with two minutes remaining. If you are unable to bring a clock or watch with you on the day, you may also ask the assessor to let you know when there are a certain number of minutes to go. However, some candidates may be put off their train of thought by this and may prefer to keep an eye on the time themselves.

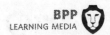

Suggested approach to the simulated exercises

There are several different approaches that you can take and indeed there is not necessarily one correct method of consulting. Many of you may have heard of several different consultation models which have been proposed by different people. You will be happy to hear that you do not need to have an in depth knowledge of the various consultation models for this assessment.

As stated before you may be faced with a variety of cases and it is unlikely that you will require every single point used in this particular consultation model. For example, you may have a case where you are required to explain a normal test result and therefore will not have an opportunity to really form a detailed management plan. On the other hand you may have a case where a patient comes to you with a new complaint, e.g. back pain, and therefore your diagnosis and management plan will be more relevant. Try to remember that this suggested consultation approach is a general guide and not every point will be relevant to each of the cases. Also, although the points are listed in a numerical order you do not need to follow this order for your scenarios. The important thing is that you have asked the relevant questions, regardless of what order you asked them in. This will become clearer as you work through the practice simulated exercises.

Suggested approach to the consultation

1. **Creating a safe environment for the patient, relative or colleague**

    This is scored in virtually all of the scenarios and is therefore something that you need to concentrate on.

    A safe environment literally means one where the patient, relative or colleague feels comfortable and is happy to open up to you. This requires thought about the physical layout of the room and about your own body language. As explained, you will have five minutes to read the brief and set up the room. There is no set rule to how the furniture should be arranged, but in general you should avoid any physical barriers between you and the patient. These barriers may be a desk or a spare chair and may act as a psychological barrier to the patient opening up to you. Therefore, if possible move the desk out

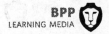

of the way so that there are no physical barriers between you and the patient. Ideally, there should be no furniture between you and the patient.

You then need to think about how to position your chair in relation to that of the patient. It is useful to have the chairs placed slightly at an angle so that you are not directly facing each other. It can be deemed quite confrontational to have your chair at a 180 degree angle to the patient's chair and can be intimidating and off-putting for the patient to have you directly in front of them. This means that you can perhaps have one chair facing straight ahead but have the other chair placed slightly to the side.

Also, you need to remember that the patient, relative or colleague may express emotion during the consultation, such as anger or may break down. Therefore you need to think about the distance you are going to have between the two chairs, ie between you and the patient. On the one hand you should allow yourself sufficient room away from the patient, relative or colleague in case they become angry as being very close may antagonise them. However, on the other hand you will need to be sufficiently close so that you are able to pass a tissue across or perhaps place a comforting hand on a shoulder if they are distressed. Do not forget however that you can adjust your position during the consultation. Therefore, if the patient, relative or colleague does become upset you can always move your chair closer if you are slightly too far away, or move it further away if you feel you are too close

You should also pay attention to your own body language during the consultation. You may naturally cross your arms when sitting, but this can look quite defensive or confrontational. Try to relax your arms by your side and lean forward slightly to show interest in what is being said. Practise various positions to see what feels comfortable for you.

Also ensure you make eye contact throughout the consultation. This will not only allow you to pick up on any non-verbal clues but will show that you are listening and interested in what they have to say. Although you may be nervous, try not to

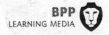

divert your gaze away especially when they are talking. This may be interpreted as you being insensitive or not listening to what they have to say.

In addition, try to maintain eye contact even if the patient, relative or colleague has looked away. This may happen when recounting a difficult or sensitive experience or feeling upset or embarrassed. Try not to let this make you feel uncomfortable and cause you to look away as well. This is likely to make the patient, relative or colleague feel even more uncomfortable and reluctant to tell you how they feel. Therefore, try to maintain eye contact at all times even if contact is broken. However, you must also be careful that you are not overly staring which will obviously be very off-putting.

A special point should be made about you remaining calm during the consultation. If you appear nervous or agitated this is likely to make the patient, relative or colleague feel uncomfortable. However, more importantly if a patient, relative or colleague is angry or annoyed during your exercise, it is important to remain calm and not raise your voice or become aggressive as you will be scored on your ability to remain calm.

2. **Introduction and opening statement**

The introduction is crucially important as it determines how at ease the patient, relative or colleague feels with you initially. You will usually be asked to call them from outside the room and thus you need to think about your approach. In some cases your brief will state whether you have seen the patient, relative or colleague before or whether they are new. It is important to be friendly and pleasant when introducing yourself. Some of you may feel comfortable shaking hands whereas some of you may simply invite the patient, relative or colleague in and ask them to sit down. If you are given the patient, relative or colleague's name in the brief however, you should use it when inviting them in. Also, if you have not seen them before you should make a point of introducing who you are and stating that you don't think you have seen them before, e.g.

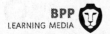

> *'Hello Mr Smith. Nice to meet you please come in and have a seat. My name is Doctor White. I don't believe we have met before?'*

This at least gives the patient, relative or colleague some idea of who you are and that you are at least intuitive and informed enough to realise that you have not met them before. It may also be the prompt they need to tell you that they have not seen you before, as they saw your colleague about the same problem, but were not happy with the advice they were given.

On the other hand it may be that they simply say, 'no we have not met before', in which case you will need to think about your next question. As mentioned before this should be an open-ended question which allows the patient, relative or colleague to tell you their story. If you used a close statement such as, 'have you have come for your test results?', you are going to create more work for yourself. This is because the patient can only reply with a 'yes' or 'no' answer. Thus it is wise to use an open-ended question as your opening statement which will encourage the full telling of their story. Useful statements to use as part of your opening sentence are:

> - *'Would you like to tell me what has brought you here today?'*
> - *'How can I help you today?'*

You can use any phrase that you feel comfortable with. However, avoid asking a question such as, 'how are you?' as you may get a difficult patient who replies with, 'well obviously I am not well as I wouldn't be here otherwise.' This is not to say that there is anything drastically wrong with this response but you may feel quite put off by this reply and is easily avoided through use of a better phrase.

3. Encourage other's contribution at appropriate points in the consultation

This involves 'active listening' which was discussed in detail earlier. This involves being silent at the appropriate points

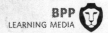

but also picking up on clues and encouraging them to talk at the right times. The key is to remember when to speak and when to listen. In general, after you have made your opening statement let the patient, relative or colleague speak until they finish. Try not to interrupt during this time. You can however use both verbal and non-verbal gestures to show that you are listening and encourage them to continue.

Examples of this would be to nod your head as you are listening or perhaps to say 'mmm' if they say something quite upsetting for them or important. The patient, relative or colleague may also pause prematurely especially if they need some encouragement from you to continue. This may because it is a difficult subject for them to discuss or perhaps because they are not sure if you are paying attention. Therefore, you may need to actively say something at this point to encourage them to continue their story. Examples of useful sentences to do so would be:

- *'That is interesting . . . tell me more.'*
- *'Mmm . . . please go on.'*
- *'I understand this is difficult for you to discuss, take your time.'*

Consequently, as a general rule, after you have introduced yourself and made your opening statement sit back and let the patient, relative or colleague talk. However, remember that some people may need a little encouragement to tell you their story and their hidden concerns. If they seem to be a little uncomfortable or hesitant in telling you the whole story, try both verbal and non-verbal gestures to help encourage them to open up.

4. **Respond to cues that lead to a deeper understanding of the problem**

This again forms part of active listening and you need to observe for cues from the actor. As stated before there is usually an underlying issue in the simulated exercise and the actor will rarely reveal everything without the correct prompting. Therefore, as the patient, relative or colleague is talking, you

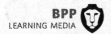

not only need to listen to what they are saying, but to pay attention to how they are behaving and how they are feeling. For example, some people may come across as nervous, either because they are speaking fast or perhaps fidgeting. Some may seem down and perhaps avoid eye contact indicating that there may be something else concerning them. Some people may give you very straightforward verbal indication of their feelings such as, 'oh I'm worried doctor.'

To gain a deeper understanding about these verbal and non-verbal clues it is important to 'reflect back' what has been said. Reflecting back is literally repeating back what the patient, relative or colleague has said to you and possibly asking for more clarification on the matter. This not only shows that you have been paying attention but also avoids any misunderstanding. Therefore you may say:

- *'You mentioned earlier that you feel you have a chest infection, what do you understand by a chest infection?'*
- *'You seem to be a little anxious today, would I be correct in saying that?'*
- *'You said earlier that you know this is something serious. What did you mean by that?'*

By asking these questions you are showing the assessors and the patient that you have picked up on the clues given to you. These clues will also help you to determine exactly what is going on and what the patient, relative or colleague is concerned about. Remember that although the actor will try to give you as many clues as they can it is your responsibility to pick up on them.

5. **Elicit appropriate details to place the complaints in a social and psychosocial context**

This section involves putting into context how the presenting complaint, no matter how straightforward and trivial it is, is affecting the patient's life and emotional well-being. For example, a young woman may have a simple dry cough but this may be affecting her life greatly if she is a singer or if she is a single mother and cannot sleep at night as a result.

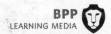

Therefore, you need to explore how the presenting complaint is affecting the patient and should get into the habit of doing so for all the cases. Even if the patient has come back to discuss a test result, you can still enquire on how the wait for this result has affected them and their loved ones. This will help you to form a clearer picture of how the patient, relative or colleague is thinking and feeling as a whole and will enable you to treat them more holistically.

Different cases will lend themselves to different psychosocial questions and you need to think of a few questions that would be pertinent to your scenario. These questions should ideally be open questions that allow the patient, relative or colleague to express how they feel and allow you to pick up on clues. It is better to ask, 'how is this affecting your sleeping?' as opposed to, 'is this affecting your sleep?' If you have a young patient who has a family you may need to ask about the financial impact of their illness if appropriate or how it is affecting their family life. If you have an elderly patient who is retired this would not be appropriate, and you may need to concentrate more on the social and psychological aspect of the illness, especially how they are managing at home. It may also be appropriate if they are suffering with a chronic or life-threatening condition to ask them if they have any religious beliefs or support that may be relevant. However, useful general questions that you can use are:

- *'How are you coping with your illness at the moment?'*
- *'What does this stop you from doing?'*
- *'How is this affecting your relationship/marriage?'*
- *'How does your illness affect your job? Are you managing to cope at work at the moment?'*
- *'How are you managing with being unwell and having three children at home?'*
- *'Who do you have at home to help you?'*
- *'Do you have any spiritual or religious beliefs? Is there someone at your church you can talk to?'*

You do not need to ask all of the questions in your role play but it is useful to ask two or three to ensure you score in the psychological, social and financial criteria. Spiritual beliefs

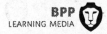

tend to become more relevant when patients are dealing with chronic conditions as opposed to acute presentations such as a fever or headache. However remember that in the assessment there is usually always some sort of psychosocial issue present, so even if it seems to be a very simple presenting complaint, make sure you ask about the impact this problem is having on their life no matter how trivial it seems.

6. **Explore the patient's understanding of their health**

    This involves exploring the patient's ideas, concerns and expectations. This is the key to revealing what exactly the patient is concerned about and perhaps if there is a hidden agenda. Unless you identify what it is that the patient is concerned about and what it is they were expecting from you, you will not be able to truly reassure the patient or address their concerns. For example, a patient may come to you with a simple headache which you diagnose as a tension headache. However, if you had not revealed that they are worried the headache is a brain tumour and they are expecting to be referred for a scan, you are unlikely to be able to truly reassure them by simply telling them it is caused by 'stress'. However, if you can now tailor your explanation incorporating their expectations you are more likely to have a successful outcome. Therefore, if you can explain why it is not a brain tumour and why a scan is not necessary they are more likely to feel reassured.

    We have previously discussed a few questions you can use to elicit the patient's ideas, concerns and expectations. You need to be very careful about how you phrase these questions as it can come across as quite abrupt if you simply ask them what they think is wrong with them. Similarly, you may elicit a response of, 'well I don't know you're the doctor'. Therefore, when asking how they think or feel, be sensitive in your approach and explain why you are asking them this. Helpful phrases to use for this purpose are:

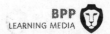

> - *'Sometimes patients have an idea as to what could be causing their symptoms. Have you had any thoughts as to what could be causing all of this?'*
> - *'You seem worried. Is there any particular thing or condition you were worried this may represent?'*
> - *'Had you had any thoughts on what you thought might happen today?'*

Also you may have picked up on clues earlier in the consultation as to what the patient thinks is wrong with them. It is useful to reflect this back to try and gain a deeper understanding of what they feel is causing their symptoms. Therefore if a patient tells you, 'it's my sinuses doctor', ask them what they mean by that. Your definition of a sinus problem may differ from the patient's so do not miss out on this vital opportunity to explore what the patient understands about their own health. There must be a reason as to why they have already given themselves a diagnosis; perhaps they have had a sinus problem before or perhaps they have read something in a magazine which they think fits their symptoms. Once you have explored what they understand about their symptoms it will become much easier to tailor your explanation and management plan to incorporate the patient's expectations.

7. **Obtain sufficient information to include or exclude likely relevant significant conditions**

    This involves taking a focused medical history to ensure you have not missed anything serious. For many of the scenarios, this will not be important as it may be that you are breaking bad news or explaining a diagnosis or test result where there is no need to take a history. However, it does seem to be a section that candidates spend a great deal of time on as they are used to taking hospital medical clerkings, where the whole emphasis of the clerking is based on the medical history and diagnosis. As stated previously, try to get out of this habit for the assessment as very little marks are given for obtaining the medical history. Also, if you spend too much time on this section you are likely to run out of time to ask about more relevant psychosocial information.

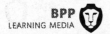

In addition, as you have now gathered the necessary psychosocial information and had an insight into how the patient is thinking and feeling it is entirely appropriate to use closed questions to take a history swiftly. Therefore you can now ask the patient quick questions to which they can only answer 'yes' or 'no'. This will help you to quickly take a history to exclude any serious medical conditions.

It is useful therefore to think about a few 'red-flag' or important symptoms for some of the common presentations, as mentioned in the 'keep to time' section. Red-flags are symptoms that may indicate to you that there is something serious going on and ruling these symptoms out will allow you to exclude any serious condition. Therefore if someone has a cough you may need to ask about smoking, shortness of breath, haemoptysis or weight loss to exclude cancer. If they are a younger patient it may be relevant to ask about wheeze, atopy or family history of asthma. These simple questions will allow you to do a quick screen and exclude any serious pathology. Other common scenarios you may be given and the red flag symptoms for those conditions are listed below:

Headache
Ask about: weight loss, visual symptoms, memory loss, pain that keeps you awake at night, early morning headaches, pain on coughing, sneezing or change in posture.

Back pain
Ask about: weight loss, fever, leg weakness, saddle anaesthesia, bladder/bowel disturbance.

Depression
Ask about: any hallucinations, psychotic symptoms or suicidal ideation.

Suspected UTI
Ask about: fever, loin pain and vomiting (to rule out pyelonephritis). Also ask about frank haematuria and urinary retention if appropriate.

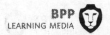

Chest pain

Ask about: shortness of breath, risk factors for cardiac disease, relation of the pain to exercise, cough, nausea, palpitations.

This list is not exhaustive but gives you an idea of the relevant questions you need to ask and reinforces the concept that it is not necessary to obtain a full medical history. This section should only take you a minute or two. Usually by the time the patient has finished telling you about their presenting complaint you have a good idea of the diagnosis is, and therefore should only need to ask a few more questions to exclude relevant conditions. Please remember that this assessment is not about taking a history or examining the patient, so do not spend too much time on this section.

8. **Choose an appropriate physical or mental assessment**

    This section is included for completeness but most of you will not be required to examine the patient. It may be appropriate when dealing with depressed or anxious presents to conduct a mental state assessment as the patient is seeking to gain some insight into how bad the situation is. Normally, you will not be required to do a physical assessment of the patient. However, you can mention at the end of your discussion that you would like to examine the patient if appropriate, as discussed previously. However, as a general rule try not to worry about this section too much as you are unlikely to be tested on it in the assessment.

9. **Make a clinically appropriate working diagnosis**

    Again, this has been included for completeness and to give your approach to the consultation some structure. However, very little marks are given for the clinical diagnosis. Some of the exercises may involve a patient who is coming to see you with a new complaint, in which case if you can come to a likely diagnosis or differential diagnosis you will gain marks. However, for some of the scenarios the diagnosis will have already been made and you might be explaining the condition, e.g. telling a patient they are asthmatic or diabetic. Remember that you may also encounter a scenario where you

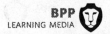

are told that certain results and investigations are negative, e.g. a patient who is tired all of the time but whose blood results are all normal. Therefore it may be more appropriate in these circumstances to not give the patient a diagnosis but perhaps to explain to them what diagnoses and conditions have been ruled out.

10. **Explain the diagnosis to the patient in appropriate language taking into account the patient's elicited beliefs**

If your scenario involves explaining the diagnosis to a patient, or perhaps explaining to them what diagnoses have been ruled out, it is important to do this in a way that the patient will understand. Therefore, try to avoid using any complicated medical terminology and use words the patient is likely to recognise, e.g. 'cancer' as opposed to 'malignancy'. It is also important to take into account the patient's ideas, concerns and expectations when explaining the diagnosis to the patient. This shows the assessors that you are taking active steps to reassure the patient and have taken their beliefs and concerns into account.

For example, you may have a 25-year-old patient who comes in to see you with a stiff neck. During the consultation you gather that the patient woke up with this pain two days ago and has no worrying features. The patient herself feels that perhaps she has slept awkwardly causing some muscle pain, however is worried it may represent arthritis. She is concerned about this particularly as her grandmother had arthritis in her later years and became severely disabled.

When explaining the diagnosis to this patient, which is simply that she has a stiff neck due to muscle spasm; it is useful to incorporate her beliefs into your explanation. You could say:

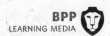

'Miss Red, after examining you today I think you are correct in saying that you are likely to have slept awkwardly causing the muscles in your neck to go into spasm. Do you understand what I mean when I say a muscle spasm?' [Let the patient answer.] 'When I touch the left side of your neck where you say the pain is the muscles feel very stiff and tender, which would fit with the diagnosis of a muscle spasm. This pain is unlikely to be due to arthritis because you are very young to have that condition and there are no features of arthritis on examination. As arthritis is a condition that affects the joints, we would expect some pain or stiffness in the area of your neck where the joints are based. Today examining you, there seems to be no problem with the small bones of the neck itself or the joints making arthritis very unlikely.'

This explains the diagnosis simply but also reassures the patient that this condition is not arthritis. Consequently, you have taken their beliefs into account during your explanation of the diagnosis to the patient. As the patient has already used the word 'arthritis' herself, it is appropriate to use it in the explanation. This is because you are reflecting back what she has said, using her words, but are also taking steps to explain to her what arthritis is. Obviously, if the patient had not mentioned arthritis at all it may not have been appropriate to use this word in your explanation as the patient may have no idea as to what it means.

You must also never assume that the patient understands what you mean. Therefore, you must take active steps to explain the diagnosis to the patient even if it seems quite simple. It is also useful to find out what exactly the patient knows or understands about the diagnosis you have given them. Some patients may be quite well informed whereas others may need a more in-depth explanation. By finding out what the patient knows already you are now showing the assessors that your communication skills are flexible and you can adapt them and tailor them to the needs of the patient. It is useful to use a general format of:

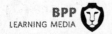

> • 'Mr X, examining you today I think you have condition
>   B (for example). Do you understand what condition B is?
>   That's right Mr X, condition B is when . . .'
> • 'Mr X, examining you today I think you have a chest infection.
>   Do you understand what I mean by a chest infection? That
>   is correct Mr X, a chest infection is when a bug gets into
>   your lungs and causes an infection. It is normally picked
>   up in the air the same way that other coughs and colds are
>   and can cause you to feel quite unwell . . .'

Try to practise explaining conditions to patients in simple words while on your medical jobs to see which phrases you feel comfortable with. These phrases are only a guide. You may have different phrases that you use to explain things to patients and some of you may prefer to use diagrams or pictures. There are several different approaches which would all be deemed suitable. The main point is to explain the diagnosis to the patient in words that they can understand ideally taking into account some of the health beliefs you have elicited previously.

11. Make an appropriate management plan

Again, very little marks will be given for this, however it is an easy place to gain marks and an area you should all feel comfortable with. Some of the simulated exercises may be straightforward where the diagnosis is clear, e.g. a viral upper respiratory tract infection. For these cases, if you are aware of the management plan then propose a clear plan for the patient, once again explaining it in terms the patient can understand.

Some of you however may encounter more complex cases or may be unsure of the diagnosis or the management. Try not to be too disheartened by this as you are unlikely to lose many marks for not getting the diagnosis and management correct. It is slightly better however if you do not know what is wrong with the patient to be honest and say so, therefore accepting your own limitations. This is preferable to taking a guess or making an absurd management plan that may cause you to lose marks. It is perfectly acceptable to tell the patient that

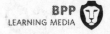

you are not sure what is causing their symptoms but you are going to conduct some further investigations to try and find out. You can also tell a patient that you would like to receive a second opinion from a senior colleague as you are unsure about how to proceed further. There is nothing wrong with doing this and indeed the assessors will appreciate the fact that you are at least being safe and realising when you are out of your depth.

12. Involve the patient in significant management decisions

The consultation within a general practice setting should be patient-centred. There is less emphasis on the doctor dictating what is right for the patient and the patient is included in making decisions on their own management. This empowers the patient giving them some degree of control over their own illness and is likely to make the patient more compliant with the management plan. As a result the assessors will be looking to see that you actively do this in your consultation.

As a result, you need to give your patient a choice in what to do and how to manage their complaint. You may also ask them beforehand if they have had any thoughts on what you should do, and this will allow you to try and take their wishes into consideration when formulating the management options. The important thing is to offer a choice and therefore you will need to suggest two or more reasonable management plans for them to choose from. For example, you may offer a patient with a viral upper respiratory tract infection the chance to come back if it worsens or perhaps a delayed prescription of antibiotics that they can use if they are not better. Useful phrases you may wish to use are:

- *'Have you had any thoughts on what you would like to do about this?'*
- *'The options we could try are to observe, wait and see if this pain goes away by itself or perhaps try some painkillers in the meantime. Which would you prefer?'*

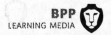

> • *'We could refer you directly to a dermatologist today. However, usually they like to know that we have tried simple things to see if they help. Therefore, we could try a steroid cream which I think would help the rash and refer you after if it does not work in about 2–3 weeks. What do you think would be best?'*

Candidates sometimes get worried that the patient may then choose an option that perhaps isn't the best option. For example, a patient who has had back pain for one week may want a physiotherapy referral which you feel is a bit premature at this stage. However, if you explain to the patient why you feel a certain option is appropriate they are usually happy to go with the option you recommend. However, it is important to give them the choice. Therefore, if you find yourself in a situation where the patient requests an option that you feel is not the most suitable, you may say to the patient:

> *'Physiotherapy is an excellent option in trying to manage lower back pain. However, as most people are pain free by six weeks the physiotherapists usually like to see patients whose pain has persisted for at least this time period. As your pain has only been there for a week now we could wait and see what happens. If the pain has not gone away in the next couple of weeks, which I expect it will do, we could refer you to the physiotherapists. However, we could also refer you now and perhaps cancel the referral if the pain gets better before then? Which would you prefer?'*

The likelihood is now that you have explained to the patient why physiotherapy may be a little premature at this stage they will be happy to wait and see. However, if they insist do try and respect the patient's decision. Fortunately, in the assessment you will find that once you have explained something adequately, the actor is quite happy to take your advice. If a patient is not happy with your management plan it is usually because you have missed a hidden agenda or have not addressed a particular concern.

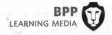

13. **When prescribing take steps to enhance concordance by exploring and responding to the patient's understanding of the treatment**

Concordance is a method which involves the patient in their treatment process, explaining to them how their medication works and why they need to take it. This is different to compliance which simply means telling a patient how to take their medication and does not take their thoughts or feelings into consideration. By improving concordance however you will ultimately improve compliance. This is because the patient will be more likely to understand their medication and therefore more likely to take it correctly.

This criterion may not be appropriate to all of the simulated exercises as it will only really be relevant if you are prescribing something for a patient, albeit a medication or a treatment. You may however, have a case where you have to explain how to use a treatment or perhaps have to deal with a patient who is not taking their medication properly. Therefore it is useful to get into the habit of making sure your patient understands how to take their medication and why they need it.

Steps you can take to improve concordance are by explaining to the patient how the medication works and why they need to take it. Patients commonly leave the doctor's surgery with medication but do not understand why they need to take it. Therefore, if you are prescribing a medication for a patient you should aim to explain to the patient:

- What the medication is for.
- The possible side effects and what they should do if this happens, e.g. do they need to stop taking it?
- How to take the medication.
- How long they need to take it for.

You should also take steps to try and improve the patient's compliance with the medication, e.g. perhaps prescribing a liquid if they have problems with tablets or a spacer with their inhaler if they have difficulties using their hands.

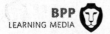

Therefore, if you have seen a patient and decided to start them on a selective serotonin reuptake inhibitor (SSRI) for their depression you may need to explain the following things to the patient:

'We have decided that an anti-depressant may be the best way to help your mood at the moment. Do you understand how anti-depressants work? (Let the patient answer.) These work by gradually allowing the body to replace the happy chemical in your body that you need in order to enjoy life. Because this is a gradual process it may take 4–6 weeks for you to see an effect. You need to take the tablet every day and if you skip days it may take even longer for the happy chemicals to build up and make you feel better. The tablets are not addictive but possible side effects include stomach upset, blurred vision or a dry mouth. The tablets may also make you feel slightly drowsy but you may have no side effects at all. If you have any side effects you should stop the tablets and consult a doctor immediately. We would suggest that you stay on the tablets for at least six months just to ensure that you are fully recovered before we stop them. However, you may need to take them for longer but we can discuss this in the future should the need arise.'

This sort of conversation is likely to ensure that the patient understands why they are on the medication and take their tablets correctly because they now understand how they work. By informing them of the side effects it also gives them a chance to discuss any concerns they have and at least ensures they do not panic if any of the side effects occur. This is more beneficial than just giving them a prescription and dictating to them that they should take one tablet a day.

Equally if a patient is not taking their existing medication correctly it is useful to reverse this procedure. Ask the patient what they understand about their medication and if they are having any difficulties in taking it, e.g. practical problems or perhaps side effects. This will allow you to address the patient's understanding about the medication and address any concerns they have.

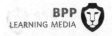

Remember you can also use this approach when you have recommended a treatment or a procedure for a patient and not just when you have prescribed a medication. For example, if you have suggested physiotherapy for a patient it is useful to ascertain they understand what physiotherapy is, that it is an ongoing process and they will need to attend a number of sessions before they see any improvement. It is surprising how many patients do not attend further physiotherapy appointments because they did not understand that they were unlikely to feel better after one session.

14. Specify the conditions and interval for follow up and review (safety net)

Safety-netting does not simply involve saying to the patient 'come back if you are not any better'. It involves giving the patient a specific time frame within which they need to return as well as the symptoms they need to look out for. Remember that general practice is the art of managing uncertainty, and as you have no access to any immediate investigations you need to ensure that you have covered all possible eventualities. Thus safety-netting is crucial. For example, you may say to the mother of a child with a viral upper respiratory tract infection who you have seen on a Friday evening:

> 'You need to see a doctor straight away if the fevers are not settling or your son should become drowsy, short of breath or develop a rash. If this does not happen but he does not seem to be back to his usual self in another week please book an appointment to see me or another doctor.'

This is informing the mother as to exactly what she needs to watch out for and is ensuring that you have not missed an important diagnosis such as meningitis or a chest infection. Had you said to the mother bring him back if he is 'unwell' it would have been very non-specific. The mother may miss vital signs which suggest her soon is severely unwell or perhaps may bring her son back to see you for a very minor symptom. Therefore, you need to be specific. Other useful phrases you may wish to use are:

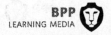

> - *'Your blood tests will take three to five days to come back. Could you make sure that you call up in seven days for the results.'*
> - *'Most people have back pain for up to six weeks. If the pain in your back lasts longer than this please come and see a doctor. However, in the meantime should you develop any limb weakness, numbness around your bottom area or problems passing water/opening your bowels please see a doctor straight away even if it is after hours.'*
> - *'I think this cough is a simple viral infection. It should clear up in about two to three weeks. However should you develop any shortness of breath, high fevers or cough up any blood please see a doctor straight away. If the cough persists beyond three weeks you will also need to come back and see us.'*

Adapt these phrases to what you feel comfortable with. Practise a few phrases every day with your patients at work. The key is to actually specify the condition or symptoms your patients need to watch out for and the time frame within which they need to come back and see you within.

15. Confirm the patient's understanding

Although this criterion is placed at the end you can use it earlier in the consultation and it is good practice to ensure that the patient understands you throughout the consultation. In the 'skills for the consultation' section the use of clarification was discussed. This is where you summarise what the patient (or relative or colleague) has said to not only let the patient know that you have been listening but to ensure that you have understood.

It is useful to use this approach after you have gained all the necessary information, ie before you make your diagnosis or explain the management. This ensures that you have understood correctly and it is useful to ensure you have the history correct well before you go on to make a plan. An example of how you may do this is:

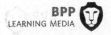

'Mrs Smith, you have come to see me today about your irritating cough. It has been going on for about a week now and you have no other worrying features. It is keeping both you and your husband awake at night and is concerning you as you are a professional singer and have a concert to perform next week. You think it is just a virus but you would like to make sure you have not got a chest infection. Is that correct?'

It is also imperative to make sure that the patient has understood the diagnosis and the management plan before they have left the room. The assessoss will be looking to make sure that you do this in every consultation. Therefore at the end of the consultation you must use a summary once again to check for understanding. It is not sufficient to simply ask if they have understood what has been discussed. Even if they say 'yes' it does not demonstrate that they have understood. Useful phrases you can use to check for understanding are:

- *'A lot has been said today. Just so that I can make sure that we have both understood each other would you like to summarise what we have discussed today?'*
- *'I would like to make sure that we have both understood each other today. If you were to go home and perhaps tell your husband what we have said today, what would you tell him?'*
- *'From what we have discussed today what do you understand? How would you explain your condition to someone else?'*

This is an excellent way to end the consultation and if possible should form part of your closing statement. After the patient has summarised everything back to you, hopefully correctly, you can simply ask them if they have any questions, hopefully to which they should answer 'no'. Don't worry if your scenario does not allow you to close the consultation in this way. However, if you are able to finish with the patient repeating back to you exactly what you have said, confirming they have understood, it is an excellent way to prove to the assessoss that you have the necessary communication skills.

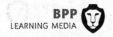

Special scenarios

This 15-part approach is straightforward when you have a patient who has a new presenting complaint and you may be able to address all 15 criteria in this type of scenario. However, as stated previously there will be cases where it is impossible to meet all of these criteria, especially when you are not required to diagnose or create a management plan. All of the scenarios however will involve the need to explore the patient's health understanding, particularly asking them about their ideas, concerns and expectations. You will also nearly always be expected to assess the effect that their presenting complaint is having on their life and emotional wellbeing, as there is usually always a psychosocial issue at hand. Therefore, you will find that points one to six in the suggested approach can be used in all of the scenarios you encounter. The assessoss will also always check that you have confirmed understanding and therefore point 15, where you ask the patient to summarise what has been discussed, will also always be relevant.

Despite this, there may be special scenarios where it is easier to use a different approach to the consultation and these will now be discussed.

Breaking bad news

Having to break bad news is a very common scenario in the simulated exercise and therefore is a situation you must feel comfortable in handling. Although there are certain aspects in the approach already discussed that are applicable to breaking bad news, there is a particular model that you might find helpful in these scenarios. This model is called the SPIKES approach and was put forward by Baile *et al.* (2000) in an oncology journal. Although the approach was designed for delivering bad news to cancer patients it can be applied to breaking bad news in any scenario. The SPIKES approach involves: Setting up, Perception, Invitation, Knowledge, Emotions, Strategy and Summary.

- Setting up: this means ensuring that your environment is suitable to break bad news to the patient. This will include ensuring that you have sufficient time and that the room is private. It should also include offering the patient the opportunity to have a friend or relative present. It may also

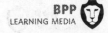

mean minimising interruptions such as closing the door or putting your phone on silent.

- **Perception:** this involves trying to find out what the patient knows (their perceptions) already. For example, was the patient already expecting bad news? Did they understand why the tests were being done and what the possible outcomes were? By finding out what the patient already knows you can adapt your explanation to take the patient's understanding and expectations into account.

- **Invitation:** this is actively having the patient's permission to break the bad news. To do this you will need to ascertain how much the patient would like to know about the diagnosis, prognosis and treatment. You may need to ask the patient, 'how much about the results would you like to know?' You may also wish to ask them if they would like the basic information about the results or whether they would like more detailed information.

- **Knowledge:** once you have established how much the patient wishes to know, you should then give the patient the necessary information in clear and simple language that they can understand. The information should be given in small segments taking into account that the patient is likely to be upset and will find it hard to take in everything you say. You may need to repeat certain pieces of information and make sure that the patient had understood.

- **Emotions:** the patient may exhibit a wide range of emotions (e.g. anger, fear, denial) so you must be able to empathise with the patient and acknowledge their feelings. This will involve active listening as well as empathic statements that show you understand the patient's reaction. For example, if a patient bursts into tears at the news, it is important to explain to the patient that you understand how upsetting this must be for them. You should also use non-verbal gestures such as touch, body language and so on where appropriate.

- **Strategy and Summary:** this involves summarising the information discussed and discussing a strategy for the future. This ensures that the patient has understood what has been said and can help the patient to understand what will happen next. This part of the consultation obviously needs to be tailored to how ready the patient is to move on. For some patients the diagnosis may come as a very big shock and they will not

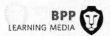

be ready to discuss how to proceed next. Your strategy may simply involve arranging a future appointment. Other patients may wish to discuss whether curative/palliative treatments were appropriate. Consequently, you may need to give them written or verbal information on what to do next and should ensure you have arranged some sort of follow up.

This approach is similar to the 15-part approach already discussed and involves: creating a safe environment, exploring the patient's ideas concerns and expectations, communicating to the patient in clear language, empathising/active listening and summarising. These are all issues that are addressed in the previous approach and are used for most scenarios.

Many of you may have your own methods for breaking bad news and do not need to follow this approach exactly. The SPIKES approach is one of many models that have been put forward for breaking bad news and it would be perfectly appropriate to use another model that you feel comfortable with, as long as you address the necessary points. However, the SPIKES approach is quite simple and as it is a mnemonic and easy to remember. However, once again use this as a guide and do not be afraid to use your own personal touches where appropriate.

Dealing with the angry or upset patient, relative or colleague

You may have a scenario where you are faced with an upset patient or relative. This may be because a mistake has been made or they may be angry due to the level of care their relative has received. These scenarios are particularly designed to see how you cope under pressure which forms part of the mark scheme. In addition to the general approach discussed, there are certain factors which you need to ensure you address. The key in these situations is to remain calm at all times and to listen to the patient or their relative even if you feel their criticisms are unfounded. It is also important to be very non-threatening in both your verbal and non-verbal language. Therefore, stay calm and seated and do not interrupt the patient or relative as they talk or shout. In addition, never raise your voice even in response to loud and threatening behaviour, as this will only antagonise the situation.

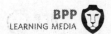

If a mistake has been made you should always be apologetic and never try to make excuses for what has happened. Empathy is paramount. You must show the assessors that you acknowledge why the patient is upset and how they must be feeling. There may be other cases however, where a relative or patient is upset for something that truly is not anyone's fault. For example, a terminally ill relative may have inevitably passed away but the family feel it was due to some sort of negligence. Here you would have a duty to empathise with how upsetting the whole scenario is for the family balancing it out with tactfully informing the relatives that this was a situation that could not have been prevented. The scenarios will obviously vary; however once you listen to the patient or their relative without interrupting and show empathy you will be able to deal with most of the scenarios.

How to cope when things go wrong

Although there may be specific scenarios in the assessment where you are expected to deal with angry patients to assess how you cope under pressure, it may be that the consultation goes wrong. As a result, what should have been a straightforward consultation ends up with an upset or annoyed patient, relative or colleague. The actors behave like real-life people and if you say something wrong or perhaps make them feel that you are not listening, there is a risk of them showing how unhappy or upset they are. This may result in something as obvious as a patient/actor telling you, 'You're not listening'. However, it may be something more subtle such as a patient reiterating the same information they have told you or saying, 'I understand doctor but . . .' They may also give you a non-verbal clue such as looking confused when you are explaining the diagnosis or looking as though they are unhappy with what you have said.

If the actor does this it usually means you have not addressed their issue or concern. Do not waste time by repeating exactly what you have said. They are unlikely to be looking unhappy because they have not heard you , it is more likely because they do not agree with it. Start again from the beginning and go through the fifteen steps we have discussed to try and identify what you have missed. It is useful to find a phrase that you can use to inform the patient that you perhaps have misunderstood each other and that you

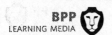

should start things over. Try to find one that you feel comfortable using yourself. Examples of such phrases are:

- *'You seem a little unhappy with the management plan we have discussed, would I be correct in saying so?'*
- *'It seems that we have misunderstood each other, perhaps we could start again?'*
- *'I am sorry that I have made you feel that way. I would really like to put the matter right so that you feel heard. Perhaps we can start again from the beginning?'*

All consultations have the potential to go wrong and even the most skilled general practitioner can tell you of situations where this has happened. However, the key is to how you get it back on track and hopefully you now have some useful tools. In addition, if you go through the steps discussed on approach the consultation thoroughly, it is very unlikely that you will put yourself in this situation.

Practice simulated exercises

In this section we will work through ten mock consultations to give you a clearer idea of the kind of topics that you will face in the assessment and an idea of how you should approach them. Obviously consultation styles differ between individuals so please remember that this is just a guide; you do not have to consult exactly as laid out in this section. However, you may find it useful to follow the approach provided for each consultation, to ensure you cover the basics. Obviously, you will have your own unique way of expressing yourself, so do not get too caught up trying to remember the phrases that we use in the role plays.

Unfortunately, although you can learn the basics about consultation skills from a book, you will not gain anything from this section if you do not practise the mock consultations. This will mean actually acting out the role of the doctor in order to practise your consultation skills, as opposed to just reading the role plays. There is also a lot to be gained by practising the role of the actor/patient. This will give you an insight into how different ways of consulting can make someone feel and how certain phrases or non verbal gestures can influence what you feel comfortable revealing.

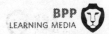

In order to truly practise these exercises, and gain the full benefit from the role plays, you will need to get together with some of your peers and act out the roles of doctor and patient. Some of you may be fortunate enough to have colleagues who are also attending the Stage 3 assessment, and it may be simple to form a practice group. However, some of you may not know anyone who is attending the assessment. Try not to worry about this; you can always ask a friend or relative to be a patient for you. There are also several websites with forums for doctors where you can look for other colleagues in your area who are sitting the assessment to practise with. Examples of these websites include doctors.net. uk and rxpgonline.com.

If possible, it is useful to have a third person in your group to act as the observer. Being an observer will give you a deeper insight into what things work well in the consultation and what things may cause the consultation to go wrong. The observer is also crucial for giving feedback to the doctor about their performance. As you can imagine the doctor and the actor will be quite involved in their roles, and therefore it is useful to have someone whose sole role is to just sit back and observe the whole consultation. However, if you are unable to have an observer in your group, the person playing the patient can also provide the feedback.

Structure of the practice consultations in this book

You are provided with two briefs for each of the mock consultations: one for the doctor and the other for the patient. There is little point practising the exercises as the doctor if you have read the patient's brief. This is because you will already know what information you need to elicit from the patient and will not be able to determine whether your normal consultation skills would have elicited the information naturally. In addition, the patient should only read their brief. The doctor's brief will give you the background to the case at hand in a summarised format. The actor's brief however will contain detailed information as to how the patient, relative or colleague should be feeling and the points that the doctor needs to elicit. It may also have information about the demeanour of the patient and non-verbal clues that they should be giving to the doctor.

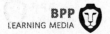

The observer, if there is one, should sit back and watch the role play assessing the consultation skills of the doctor. They should take notes on the performance of the doctor during the scenario, and give the doctor feedback as to how they have done. They could also score the doctor based on the mark scheme provided earlier. It is useful if the observer has read both the patient's and doctor's briefs before beginning the mock consultation. This allows them to determine what information the doctor knew initially and what information the doctor needed to elicit during the consultation. The observer can then look out for the exact skills that were used by the doctor to reveal this information from the patient. Also, as they are aware of what information the patient should be revealing and what clues they should be giving the doctor, it will also help them ascertain if this information was missed by the doctor and why.

The patient, relative or colleague should also be taking mental notes during the scenario, thinking about how the doctor has made them feel and the things that were done well in addition to the things that the doctor could improve on. Therefore, both the patient and the observer will be expected to give the doctor feedback at the end of the consultation.

How to give feedback

The feedback you give yourself is as important as as the feedback you receive from the pretend patient, relative or colleague and the observer. Therefore, although your colleagues will be giving you feedback on your performance, it is useful to comment on how you think the consultation went. When giving feedback you should always start with the positive comments first, ie what things went well, and leave the negative comments until later. This is because if you start with the negative comments, you are unlikely to remember any of the things you did well and feel quite defeated. The feedback should be done in three ways:

Feedback from the doctor
• What they think went well and perhaps what did not go so well and why? What they would do differently the next time and why?

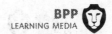

Feedback from the patient/relative/colleague

- How they felt as a patient e.g. did the doctor make them feel comfortable? Did they feel listened to? Did they have a caring manner? Would they want to see that doctor again?
- What did the doctor do well? What could they improve on? What information did they miss and what could they have done to have gained that information? Remember that in the exam these comments from the actors may be used to mark your performance overall.

Feedback from the observer

- Essentially all the above observations e.g. what they think the doctor did well and why, and what could have been improved.
- Did the doctor stay calm and composed?

Proposed mark scheme

In the practice exercises the formal mark scheme (as previously discussed), can be used to analyse the consultations and give feedback. Although you may feel that if you have gained all the information on the actor's brief you have done well, there is always room for improvement and this may not necessarily be the case. For example, although you may have elicited all the necessary information from the patient's brief, your manner or the way you phrase your words may need some adjustment. Therefore, it is useful to have a structured approach to looking at your own consultation to identify the exact areas that need improvement.

This exam is about continually relating back to the mark scheme and showing the assessors that you have clearly achieved the necessary criteria. In your practice consultations however, you may find that your colleagues are more willing to reveal the information as the patient, or that the observers mark you less harshly than real assessors. Therefore, do not aim to simply take all the information from the actor's brief; this may not be enough to pass. Try to ensure that you tick all the relevant boxes on the mark sheet. However, do try to remember that not all the points will be relevant to each consultation used.

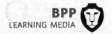

The mark scheme you may wish to use for the mock consultations is shown below. Please note that for simplicity, a number of points have been combined regarding making an appropriate diagnosis and explaining the diagnosis to the patient. The points regarding making an appropriate management plan and involving the patient in the management decision have also been combined. The mark scheme below only has 13 points as opposed to the mark scheme discussed earlier which had 15 points. To help you make the most of the practical exercises in this chapter you can download a blank version of the mark scheme below from www.bpp.com/freehealthresources

1.	Creating a safe environment for the patient	Ensuring there are no obstacles between the doctor and the patient. Are the chairs placed at an appropriate distance? Remaining calm if a patient gets annoyed or aggravated. Remaining seated if a patient is standing and aggressive.
2.	Introduction and opening statement	Introducing yourself to the patient and the use of open-ended questions. e.g. *'Hello Mrs Red I don't think we have met before? I am Dr White.'* *'Would you like to tell me what has brought you here today?'*
3.	Encourage the patient's contribution at appropriate points in the consultation	Showing the patient that you are listening and also encouraging the patient to tell you their story. e.g. nodding your head during the consultation and making appropriate eye contact. Also use of verbal gestures such as *' That's interesting please tell me more.'* *'Hmm . . . I see.'*
4.	Respond to cues that lead to a deeper understanding of the problem	Picking up on verbal and non-verbal clues given to you by the patient and trying to explore these in more detail. e.g. *'You seem anxious?'* *'You seem a little down today?'* Also reflecting the patient's words back. *'You said earlier you thought you had a sinus problem. What did you mean by that?'*

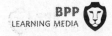

5.	Elicit appropriate details to place the complaints in a social and psychosocial context.	Trying to understand how the presenting complaint is affecting the patient as a whole. e.g. *'How is this affecting your home life?'* *'Who is at home with you?'* *'Do you have any help with your children?'* *'What does this stop you from doing?'*
6.	Explore the patient's health understanding	Exploring the patient's ideas, concerns and expectations e.g. *'Did you have any ideas as to what could be causing all of this?'* *'What is your main concern regarding this?'* *'Did you have any ideas on how I would be able to help you today?'*
7.	Obtain sufficient information to include or exclude likely relevant significant conditions	Appropriate use of questions, including closed questions to try and come to a diagnosis. A focused history relevant to the problem, e.g. red flag symptoms or a relevant systems review.
8.	Choose an appropriate physical or mental examination	Likely to not be relevant in the exam. However in certain scenarios you may gain a mark if you mention that you would examine the patient under the appropriate conditions, e.g. in another room at the end of the consultation.
9.	Make a clinically appropriate working diagnosis / explain the diagnosis to the patient in appropriate language taking into account the patient's elicited beliefs.	Makes an appropriate diagnosis to the presenting complaint (however little marks will be given for this). Uses non medical jargon to explain the diagnosis to the patient. Using the patient's own words. e.g. *' infection in your bladder'* versus *'UTI'*. *'Remember when you said you thought you had a chest infection. Earlier you said you were worried about this lump being cancer . . . I do not think it is cancer because . . .'*

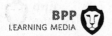

10.	Make an appropriate management plan/ involve the patient in significant management decisions.	Again little marks are given for the details of the management plan. The plan should be sensible however and appropriate for the diagnosis. It is important to involve the patient in the decisions made about their care e.g. *'The options are A when . . . Or B when . . . Which one would you like to try?'* *'Have you had any thoughts on what you would like to do?'*
11.	When prescribing take steps to enhance concordance by exploring and responding to the patient's understanding of the treatment.	Attempting to explain to a patient the details about a treatment so that they understand this treatment better and are more likely to comply. e.g. *'We have decided to prescribe A. A works by . . . Common side effects you may experience are . . . and if you do not take it daily it may not work . . . '* *'We have decided to send you for physiotherapy . . . this will involve having to do some strengthening exercises for your knee . . . this will involve you having to have weekly sessions . . . and it may take a while before you notice an effect . . .'*
12.	Specify the conditions and interval for follow up and review (safety net)	Ensuring that the worst does not happen and making sure you have a plan if your diagnosis is wrong or things worsen. e.g. *'If you should experience . . . please come back and see me in . . . days.'*
13.	Confirm the patient's understanding	Taking active steps to ensure that the patient has understood what you have said e.g. *'If you were to go and tell a friend what we have discussed today what would you say?'* *'Just to ensure that we have both understood each other would you like to summarise what has been said today?'*

Once again try to remember that all the points may not may relevant for each case. For example, there may be cases where you are clearly told that you do not need to examine the patient or cases where you do not prescribe a treatment and therefore points 8 and 13 will be redundant. Each case will differ as in the exam, so do not get worried if you cannot get all the points for each case, there are few cases that will allow you to do so.

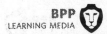

As some of the practice consultations involve explaining breaking bad news you may wish to use the SPIKES approach to mark your colleagues (as discussed previously).

Practise to time

It is useful to get into the habit of practising the mock consultations to time. This way you will develop a feel for how long you will have on the actual day and get into the habit of becoming more time-efficient in your consultations. As mentioned before, many candidates spend far too long taking medical histories and this is an area where most of you will need to concentrate on. Try not to worry if you run overtime in the first few consultations; this is to be expected. As you practise you will find that you become more familiar with what questions are relevant and your consultations will become smoother. It is not easy going from the routine of taking very long detailed hospital clerkings to a focussed 20-minute general practice consultation. Obviously, some of you in the OSCE group may have only ten minutes, and you need to find out in advance how much time you have.

For the purpose of this book the mock consultations given are perfectly achievable in 15 minutes. It is good practice for those who have 20 minutes to try and achieve the task in this shorter time, as during the assessment day nerves and actually having a real actor will extend the time slightly. For those of you doing the ten-minute OSCE, the cases discussed here will be more detailed than the ones you will be provided with on the day. Therefore if you can achieve all the relevant information in 15 minutes you will have no problems achieving less information in the ten minutes you will be given. We have tried to achieve a compromise for both types of candidates.

Once again, we advise that you allow yourself five minutes to read the doctor's brief, make notes and arrange the room how you see fit. This is what will happen on the actual exam day. The actor playing the patient, relative or colleague may wish to take some more time to read their brief and it is a good idea for the observer to also read both briefs to gain a better understanding into the case. There is no set time on how long you should spend giving feedback. Some cases may have been quite difficult for the doctor and may generate a lot of discussion. However, for cases

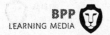

that were simpler, try to spend at least ten minutes giving detailed feedback, and not gloss over the case as it all seemed to have gone well. There is always room for improvement.

Practise, practise, practise

There are ten mock consultations for you to go through. As stated before, please do not simply read these through. Practise them with your colleagues as we have suggested previously, preferably with both a patient, relative or colleague and an observer. The first five consultations are discussed in great detail and example phrases are given. This is simply to help you if you become stuck during the consultation. However, if you used different phrases to elicit the information this is absolutely fine. Please do not be afraid to bring your own unique style to the consultation.

The last five consultations are discussed in less detail, as hopefully you will have developed a feel for how they should be approached. We simply give a check-list for these consultations to ensure that you covered the relevant points.

However, please do not stop practising after these ten consultations. You can always get together and make up your own role plays with your colleagues or practise with your every day patients, their relatives or your work colleagues. There are also different courses that you can attend which may be beneficial. The key is to constantly practise your consultation skills so that it becomes natural to you by the day of the assessment.

Good luck and happy role-playing.

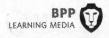

Mock Consultation 1

Doctor's brief

Mrs Benjamin, a 33-year-old lady, is coming to see you today about her weight. You have never met her before. She saw one of your colleagues two weeks ago, as she did not understand why she had gained so much weight over the last year. She had told your colleague that she had gained over three stone this year alone, and had a BMI of 33 when last checked. Your colleague had arranged some blood tests at the time; including liver function tests, a full blood count, a fasting glucose and a thyroid function test. They also arranged a 24-hour urinary cortisol excretion test to exclude Cushing's disease. All the results came back as normal and the patient was told that there was no medical cause for the weight gain.

The patient has come to you today for a second opinion as she is still gaining weight and does not understand why. There is no need to repeat the blood tests or examine the patient again.

You have 10 minutes to complete this task.

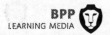

Use this space for your pre-consultation notes.

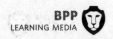

Mock Consultation 1

Patient's brief – *Do not read if you are playing the role of the doctor*

> You are Mrs. Benjamin, a 33-year-old lady, who is coming to see another GP for a second opinion. You have never met this GP before. You have gained three stone in the past year alone and are clinically obese. You are convinced there is some sort of medical reason for the weight gain; however your blood and urine tests two weeks ago have excluded this. You were told this by the GP you had seen, however you are still not convinced, and are worried as you are still gaining weight.

Information unknown to the doctor

You are having relationship problems at the moment. You have had two children (aged three and five) and are completely rushed off your feet. You started to gain weight after the birth of your children and have not been able to shift it, especially as you have little time to exercise. You are not working at the moment as you are a full time mother and are feeling quite bored and unfulfilled. Your partner is at work all the time and you are left at home alone causing you to feel very lonely. As a result you have been comfort eating and this is causing you to gain even more weight. Your partner has started to make comments about your appearance calling you 'fat' and 'podgy' and this is making you feel even more unhappy about yourself. As a result you are eating even more.

You are aware of what is causing your weight gain but are in denial about the situation as you are embarrassed to reveal what is really going on. You are also very frightened due to the impact being obese may have on your health. As a result you are worried that you may not live to see your children grow up. You will only reveal this information, however, if the doctor is sympathetic and allows you to talk about your fears. You need a lot of encouragement from the doctor to reveal what is going on.

At first you come across as aggressive because you are quite upset that no one can tell you why you are gaining weight. You are also obviously very sensitive about your weight. If the doctor tries to tell

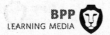

you immediately that it must be your lifestyle causing the weight gain, you become even angrier. However, if the doctor listens to you and is not judgemental, you begin to become more relaxed and will accept that perhaps it is due to your eating patterns and lack of exercise. You will then also accept any suggestions the doctor makes to you on how to lose weight and agree to lifestyle changes. However, if the doctor does not make you feel comfortable, you make constant excuses as to why you cannot exercise and deny that you comfort eat.

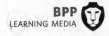

Mock Consultation 1

Information from brief

Things you may have picked up from the brief are:

Mrs Benjamin a 33-year-old lady

This is a relatively young patient who is married. Therefore, it may be important to ask her about her relationship with her husband when assessing the psychosocial impact of her presenting complaint. It may also be relevant to ask her whether she has any children. As she is of working age you may also need to ask her about her occupation and whether she is working at the moment.

Is coming to see you about her weight

What are her ideas, concerns and expectations around her weight? How could weight gain affect a person as a whole?

You have never met her before

Therefore it will be important to do a proper introduction and make her feel comfortable as this is the first time you are meeting her. You may need to do a little extra work to make her feel comfortable.

She saw one of your colleagues two weeks ago, as she did not understand why she had gained so much weight over the last year

If she has seen one of your colleagues about this why is she coming to see you? What did your colleague say to her? Could it be that they did not explain things properly? Could it be that she is unhappy with their diagnosis? Could there be a hidden agenda or does she really not understand why she has gained the weight? What is concerning her about this weight gain?

She had told your colleague that she had gained over three stone this year alone, and had a BMI of 33 when last checked by your colleague

She has gained a large amount of weight and therefore it is reasonable for her to be concerned about this. Her BMI is telling you that she

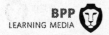

is clinically obese and gives you an idea of how heavy she is at this time. What issues could arise from someone being obese?

All the results came back as normal and she was told that there was no medical cause for the weight gain

We are told in the earlier paragraph that a wide range of tests have been requested, all of which have come back as normal. Therefore, there is no medical cause for this weight gain. Thus, you need to explore other causes and be thinking of what the other causes could be? Could she possible be depressed? Does she have a poor diet or lifestyle? If so why is this? Can she afford healthy eating? Can she afford the gym? What things could be causing this weight gain?

She has come to you today for a second opinion as she is still gaining weight and does not understand why. There is no need to examine the patient or repeat the tests again

Her presenting complaint is that she allegedly wants a second opinion as to whether there could be a medical cause for her weight gain. However, we know there is usually another psychosocial aspect to the case. Therefore we need to ensure we address this and try to explore the issues. As the brief states that we do not need to examine or repeat the tests again we need to use other skills to reassure the patient. We should also pay attention to the brief and not waste valuable time offering to re-examine the patient or repeat the tests again.

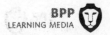

Mock Consultation 1

Suggested approach to the consultation by the doctor

1. **Creating a safe environment for the patient**

   Here you need to ensure that the furniture was correctly arranged and you were an appropriate distance from the patient. This means that you made sure there were no obstacles between you and the patient and that you were sufficiently close to the patient to offer a comforting hand or tissue if she became distressed. You should have also ensured that your chair was at a comfortable angle from the patient. This should be in a position where you could observe her demeanour comfortably and maintain eye contact and ideally should not be directly facing the patient as this can be awkward for both of you.

   You should have also monitored your own body-language and ensured that you were not defensive or looked distracted while she was talking. The patient was told to come across as aggravated initially and during this time you should have remained calm and allowed her to talk without interrupting. You should have also ensured that you kept a calm tone and did not show your frustrations when the patient was initially quite difficult.

2. **Introduction and opening statement**

   You should have greeted the patient and explained who you were. Remember the patient has never met you before and you should have tried to make her feel comfortable by introducing yourself. You were also given the patient's name in the brief and you should ideally have used this when greeting the patient.

   You should have also used an open question for your opening statement. For example, did you ask the patient what had brought her to you today and allowed her to give you a detailed answer? Or did you use a closed question and ask her if she had come about her weight? An example, of an appropriate introduction and opening statement is:

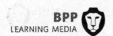

> 'Hello Mrs Benjamin, it's lovely to meet you. Please have a seat. My name is Doctor X. I don't believe we have met before? Would you like to tell me a little bit about what has brought you here today?'

Some of you may have commented on the fact that she had seen your colleague before in your opening statement.

> 'Hello Mrs Benjamin, it's lovely to meet you. Please have a seat. My name is Doctor X. I don't believe we have met before? I think you saw my colleague previously. How can I help today?'

The patient may then have revealed to you what she had seen your colleague about and what had happened during that consultation. It is important to try to establish what your colleague had told her during that consultation and also her understanding of why the tests had been requested. If she did not volunteer this information straight away it would have been important to ask her about this later once she had finished telling you why she was here today.

3. **Encourage the patient's contribution at appropriate points in the consultation**
    This may have involved maintaining eye contact throughout the consultation or nodding appropriately to show the patient you were listening. The patient should have shown you that they were uncomfortable telling you what was really going on and you should have encouraged the patient to continue what she was saying, for example:

> - 'I can understand this is a sensitive subject to discuss. Take your time.'
> - 'Please go on.'

4. **Respond to cues that lead to a deeper understanding of the problem**
    In this scenario the patient may have been quite aggressive at first; coming across as quite annoyed that no one could find out what was wrong with her.

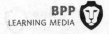

> 'Yes doctor, well I've been to see your colleague and he claims there is nothing wrong with me (said sarcastically). However, I know my body and I know that there is something causing me to gain this weight. I have not done anything different in the past year so I know there is no reason why I should be gaining this weight.'

This would allow you to reflect back how she is coming across and what she has said to try and gain a deeper understanding:

- 'You seem quite concerned about this weight gain and angry that you have been told there is nothing wrong medically. Would I be correct in saying so?'
- 'You said that you have not done anything different in the past year. What did you mean by that?'

The first statement may then allow the patient to tell you that they are angry and the reasons behind it providing you with a deeper insight into how she is feeling. By showing the patient that you have picked up on her anger it may also help to calm her down. The second statement however may be met with the response:

> 'Well doctor I have been eating exactly the same things and still not doing any exercise so I don't see what is so different.'

This could obviously then allow you to pick up on this clue she is giving you and gently introduce the subject about diet and exercise and find out what her eating and lifestyle habits were, for example:

> 'When you say you have been eating the same things what did you mean by that? What sort of things do you eat?'

The patient may then reply with:

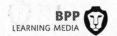

> *'Well I do tend to "pick" at things especially if I'm bored or upset. But I've always done that doctor so why would it mean I am suddenly gaining weight now?'*

Thus you have elicited the information that she comfort eats by picking up on simple clues that the patient has given you. You now have a deeper understanding of the problem.

5. **Elicit appropriate details to place the complaints in a social and psychosocial context**
   This is the key to this case and therefore you need to have ensured that you have asked the patient what effect this weight gain has had on her. To do this you will also need to find a little bit about this patient's background.

> * *'Are you working at the moment?'*
> * *'Do you have any children?'*
> * *'How is this weight gain affecting your life at the moment? Does it stop you from doing anything you want to do?'*
> * *'Has your weight gain affected your relationship? How has your husband responded to your sudden gain in weight?'*

The patient may then respond to these questions by saying:

> *'No, I am not working at the moment. I have no time to work as I have two kids to look after and my husband is never at home. I guess my weight has not stopped me from doing anything as I can't afford it to. I have to rush around looking after the kids. As for my husband, well to be honest he hasn't been the greatest . . .'*

The patient may then stop there as she is reluctant to tell you more. You may need to use your skills to encourage the patient to continue, you could say, for example:

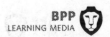

- *'He hasn't been the greatest?' (pausing after to let the patient continue)*
- *'What did you mean when you said your husband hasn't been the greatest?'*

The patient may be encouraged to reveal that, since becoming overweight her husband has been calling her names, thereby making her feel more depressed and dependent on comfort eating.

6. **Explore the patient's health understanding**
Here you need to explore the patient's ideas, concerns and expectations. Therefore you may wish to ask.

- *'You have mentioned that you know for sure that there is something going on that is causing you to gain weight. Have you had any ideas on what could be the problem?'*
- *'What is concerning you most about this weight gain?'*
- *'Do you have any ideas on how I could help you today?'*

The patient may then reply with:

'Well I know I have had two kids and I have never been skinny. But I am worried I could have an underactive thyroid because my mother had that. She felt unwell for ages and no one picked it up. She had lots of health problems because of her weight and I don't want to end up with similar problems. You know, you see it on television all the time, people who are too fat to get out the house or who get all sorts of problems. I've got two kids, doctor. I can't afford to get so fat that I won't be around to see them grow up.'

By exploring the patient's concerns you have now elicited the key information from the brief; the patient is concerned she has an underactive thyroid and, in view of her mother's condition, is concerned that her weight problem may be hereditary.

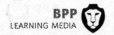

7. **Obtain sufficient information to include or exclude likely relevant significant conditions**

    This scenario does not require you to rule out a medical cause for her obesity. The brief states it has already been done. However, if you suspect that perhaps she may be depressed or that she may have a poor diet causing her weight gain, you could ask a further question to explore this (if you have the time to do so).

    - 'Mrs Benjamin, you said earlier that you tend to pick at things and comfort-eat. Tell me what a typical day is like for you. What do you normally eat?'
    - 'You mentioned that you are extremely busy with two young children at home. It must be extremely difficult therefore to exercise. Do you havet any free time to do any physical activities?'
    - 'You mentioned that your husband has not been very supportive lately and calls you names. I could imagine that that is very upsetting. Does it cause you to comfort-eat more?'

    The patient may then reply:

    - 'Well, I have a normal breakfast, like toast with jam as that's what the kids have. I skip lunch regularly as I don't have time. So before I go and pick up my older child I might have some tea and biscuits or a chocolate bar. Dinner time I usually just have what the kids eat, like chips or pizza. Most of the time however, I end up eating theirs as they can't finish it. If I'm bored however I tend to pick at chocolate biscuits. They make me feel better.'
    - 'No, I have no time to exercise at all. I am always tidying up and running after my little ones. Surely that is exercise enough? As for my husband . . . well yes, I must admit his comments make me feel worse. I just think what's the point? He thinks I'm fat so I might as well continue eating.'

    Obviously, at this point in time you now have tremendous insight into what is causing this patient's weight gain. You are also aware of how this affects her and the possible obstacles

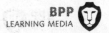

she may face in trying to lose weight. You have now nearly gained all the information from the patient's brief.

8. **Choose an appropriate physical or mental examination**
    The brief says that you do not need to examine this patient so this point is not relevant. For those of you who may be wondering if the patient was perhaps depressed, it would have been appropriate to do a mental state examination in your head as the patient was talking. However, you do not need to reveal to the assessors that you have done so.

9. **Make a clinically appropriate working diagnosis / explain the diagnosis to the patient in appropriate language taking into account the patient's elicited beliefs**
    Although you are not actually coming to a medical diagnosis you do have some idea what is causing her weight gain. Thus it would be appropriate in this case to mention this to the patient as the 'diagnosis.' You obviously need to be very careful in your approach as the patient is very sensitive about this subject. You should also make sure that you speak in simple jargon-free language and take her beliefs into account when explaining the matter to her.

'You said earlier that you were worried that you had an "underactive thyroid" causing your weight gain. The blood tests we did actually checked whether your thyroid was working and everything seems to be okay. It is very unlikely that these blood tests are wrong. Naturally, you are very worried about what will happen if you keep gaining weight and we do need to try and figure out what is causing the weight gain. Listening to what you have told me it seems that you are very busy at the moment and this causes you to grab food on the go. This may mean you eat the wrong things. Also, because you are so busy you do not get time to do any exercise. Although running after your children is obviously very tiring, unfortunately it will not burn enough calories to help you to lose weight. Finally, it seems that you are quite unhappy at the moment and are comfort-eating, perhaps eating the wrong things. I have a feeling that this may be contributing to your weight gain. What do you think?'

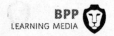

Hopefully if you have been empathic and listened to the patient she will agree with this.

10. **Make an appropriate management plan / involve the patient in significant management decisions**

Your management plan may vary. It may vary from trying to give her counselling or help in her relationship or referring her to a dietician. It doesn't really matter what you suggest as long as you involve her in the making these decisions and give her the option to choose. Ideally it would be nice to ask her how she feels you could help.

> *'It is obviously a very difficult time for you right now. Have you had any ideas on how I could help you?'*

The patient may then ask you to give her a diet plan or perhaps an anti-obesity drug or may ask you for advice. Obviously, you could also give her various suggestions.

> *'I think we have agreed that your eating patterns and lifestyle at the moment may be contributing to you gaining weight. Obviously, I fully appreciate that it is difficult for you right now to exercise as you have a busy lifestyle. Is there a possibility you could go out for a walk with your youngest child, even for half an hour, while the older one is at school? Or maybe a family member could look after your children for an hour so that you could perhaps go for a walk or go for a swim? If this is not possible perhaps we could try to address your eating habits. I could refer you to a dietician to give you some advice on what to eat or give you a medication to help you lose weight? We could also refer you to someone to talk about how you feel? Maybe by talking about your feelings you may find other ways of coping with how you feel other than eating? What do you think?'*

The patient may then reply that perhaps she could find half an hour a day to go for a walk and would like to see a dietician and a counsellor. It doesn't really matter what the patient decides to do as long as you have given her the choice and it is an informed decision that she is making.

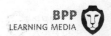

11. **When prescribing take steps to enhance concordance by exploring and responding to the patient's understanding of the treatment**
This would only be appropriate if you were going to prescribe an anti-obesity drug. However, the patient brief states that she opts for lifestyle advice so this will not be relevant.

12. **Specify the conditions and interval for follow up and review (safety net)**
In this case you may wish to see the patient again to give her some moral support and monitor her weight loss. In terms of safety-netting this would be more important with regards to her mood. As she is going through a tough time at the moment you may wish to ask her to come back if her mood deteriorates or things become worse at home.

> 'Shall we agree a date to review you again and see how you are getting on with the diet plan? I think we should see you in a month to see how you are getting on. What do you think? Obviously, I understand that it is a really stressful time for you at the moment, so I would really like you to come back immediately if things get bad and you feel that you cannot cope at home. Would that be okay?'

13. **Confirm the patient's understanding**
Ensure the patient understood everything you said by asking them to summarise your statements:

> 'Just so I can make sure we have both understood each other today could you please summarise what we have said today and what we are going to do?'

The patient should hopefully reiterate what has been said in the consultation.

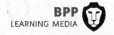

> *'Yes doctor. We have agreed that it is my diet and lifestyle that has caused me to gain weight and we will try to address that. You are referring me to a dietician and I will try and find time to do some simple activities like walking. You are also referring me to a counsellor as you think talking about the problems I am having may help me to stop comfort-eating. You would like to see me again in a month to see how I am progressing, however you would like me to see you straight away if things get really bad at home.'*

You can then simply say to the patient, 'Yes that is correct. Do you have any questions?' To which the patient should hopefully say 'no' and you can end the consultation.

Notes

As stated before this is just one suggested approach you could take to the consultation. Therefore do not worry if you didn't phrase your sentences in the exact same way as this example. This is not the only model answer but is here to give you an idea on how you can approach the situation, or to give you some useful phrases if you found certain points difficult. Also, remember that in your scenario your actor may have not given you all the clues so don't worry if certain points were not raised. Finally, do not panic if you had a different management plan as the consultation could have produced different outcomes depending on how the actor guided you. You will not be marked on your management plan in the assessment; merely on whether you gave the patient a choice and an opportunity to be involved in her own management.

If the patient became quite annoyed initially and refused to give you any information on what was going on, try to figure out why that was? Was it because you immediately assumed that she must be eating poorly and doing no exercise and started to give her advice without exploring how she felt? The patient was told specifically to become quite upset and defensive if the doctor immediately gave her solutions to her weight gain without trying to understand how it was affecting her. Maybe it was because you were taken aback when she was aggressive about your previous colleague not being able to establish what was wrong with her.

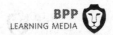

As a result you may have then gone into great detail about the blood tests being normal to try and reassure her and defend your colleague. If you did this you have obviously not elicited her concerns and have therefore missed the hidden agenda.

If your consultation went badly try to replay that part of the consultation changing the way you asked or phrased your questions. Try and see how perhaps addressing things in a different way can change the whole outcome of the consultation. If this is difficult for you, ask your colleagues for ideas as to how you could have approached things differently and what you could have said differently, and then try putting these changes into practice.

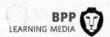

Mock Consultation 2

Doctor's brief

You are working in general practice. Ms Cathy Bowen has booked an appointment to discuss her seven-year-old daughter Megan. She has not brought Megan to the appointment today and has come alone. She is concerned about her behaviour and feels she is being very withdrawn. You have seen Megan a few times before and she has always seemed like a happy child to you. She has no relevant past medical history of note and has achieved all her developmental milestones normally. She is however an only child, and as her mother is also your patient, you are aware that her relationship with Megan's father broke-up recently. There are no child protection concerns and you have no reason to suspect that anything untoward has happened to Megan.

You have 10 minutes to complete this task.

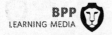

Use this space for your pre-consultation notes.

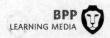

Mock Consultation 2

Patient's brief – *Do not read if you are playing the role of the doctor*

> You are Ms Cathy Bowen and have a seven-year-old daughter called Megan. She is your only child from your relationship with her father which broke-up about two months ago.

Information unknown to the doctor

Megan has always been a happy child; however since the relationship break-up with her father she has become quiet and withdrawn. You suspect that she is not coping well with suddenly not having her father around. You are feeling guilty and embarrassed as it was an affair on your part that caused the relationship to end. You feel that Megan's moods are your fault, as you should have never had the affair. To make things worse, the gentleman you were having the affair with has also left you, and you are feeling very alone.

Your parents separated as a child and you did not handle it well. You did not speak to anyone and as a result became a very angry teenager and ended up with the wrong crowd. You did not finish school due to this. You are extremely anxious that this will happen to Megan.

In addition, your ex-partner has been accusing you of being a bad mother and is threatening to apply for sole custody of Megan. You want Megan to get help, but are afraid of your ex-partner finding out about her problems and using this as a reason to prove you are an unfit mother.

You are therefore reluctant to allow the doctor to refer Megan to speak to anyone, and do not want her school contacted. However, if the doctor reveals that you are worried about your ex-partner taking Megan away and reassures you that you are not a bad mother, you become accepting for Megan to get help.

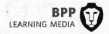

You are also secretly not coping with the break-up and this is a cry for help. You are not sleeping well or eating well and are tearful all the time. You think you may be depressed. If the doctor picks up on your depression, and has been sensitive to how you feel, you are open to any suggestions they can give you on how to help your mood.

Initially, when you go into the consultation, you just seem like an anxious parent and give off little non-verbal clues about your depression. However, as you begin to talk more about the break-up with your ex-partner you become very down and show the doctor that this is obviously a difficult subject for you.

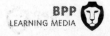

Mock Consultation 2

Information from brief

Things you may have picked up from the brief are:

Ms Bowen has booked an appointment to discuss her seven-year-old daughter Megan. She has not bought Megan to the appointment today and has come alone

Why has the mother come without Megan? Are there things she wants to discuss that she does not want Megan to hear? As her name is Ms Bowen it implies that she is not married. What is her relationship status at the moment? Is she a single mother? Is Megan's father around?

She is concerned about her behaviour and feels she is being very withdrawn

Megan is only seven years old. What could be going on that would cause Megan to be withdrawn. Is there something happening at school? Is there an issue in her home life? What does her mother mean by 'withdrawn?'

You have seen Megan a few times before and she has always seemed like a happy child to you

You know Megan and therefore probably know her mother as well. As Megan has always seemed happy to you what has happened suddenly to change this? Obviously if Megan has suddenly changed in her behaviour this is worrying.

She has not relevant past medical history of note and has achieved all her developmental milestones normally

This is telling you that Megan is unlikely to have any medical reason causing her personality change. Therefore it is likely to be a psychosocial issue.

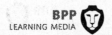

She is however an only child, and as her mother is also your patient, you are aware that she has recently broken-up with Megan's father

Is Megan being an only child relevant? Does she have anyone to talk to if she is an only child? As she is an only child you are unlikely to need to enquire about if any siblings have been affected by this break-up. Could the recent break-up of her parents be the reason for Megan's behaviour? Could it also be due to something else that perhaps her mother is unaware of or reluctant to tell you about?

There are no child protection concerns and you have no reason to suspect that anything untoward has happened to Megan

This is simply telling you that there is no need to suspect that there are any underhand reasons why Megan may be withdrawn, such as sexual abuse. It is also telling you that you do not have any reasons to worry about her mother's parenting. Therefore although you may wish to exclude this in real life there is no need to do so in this case.

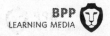

Mock Consultation 2

Suggested approach to the consultation by the doctor

1. **Creating a safe environment for the patient**

   Here you need to ensure that the furniture is carefully arranged as this is likely to be a delicate consultation. Her mother is obviously quite worried and has recently broken-up with her partner. Therefore there is the potential for her to become upset or tearful and you need to be in a suitable position to reach out to comfort her if this should happen. You should have also ensured that your chair was at a comfortable angle from the patient. This should be in a position where you could observe her demeanour comfortably and maintain eye contact, however ideally should not be directly facing the patient as this can be awkward for both of you.

   As this may be a delicate subject, and one that the mother may find difficult to talk about, you should have paid close attention to your body language and manner. Therefore, you should have tried to keep a very soft and sympathetic tone throughout the consultation to make Ms Bowen feel comfortable. You should have also maintained eye contact throughout the consultation to reassure the patient that you were listening.

2. **Introduction and opening statement**

   You should have greeted the patient and invited her in. As it is implied that you know the patient you may have addressed her by her first name. You may have still called her 'Ms Bowen', which is acceptable, but may be slightly formal under the circumstances.

   You ideally should have used an open question for your opening statement although you are told why she is coming to see you in the brief. This will allow her to give you as much information as possible and may give you some non-verbal clues as to what is going on. For example, she may have seemed upset or anxious when telling you why she was there. It would have not been appropriate to ask her if she was here because she was concerned about Megan, although you are told this in the brief. You could however have asked

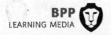

how Megan was as this would not lead onto a 'yes' or 'no' answer.

Examples of an appropriate introduction and opening statement would be:

- *'Hi Cathy please come in. Nice to see you again. Have a seat. How are you and Megan?'*
- *'Hi Cathy. How are you? Have a seat. How can I help you today?'*

3. **Encourage the patient's contribution at appropriate points in the consultation**
   This may have involved maintaining eye contact throughout the consultation or nodding appropriately to show the patient you were listening. The actor may have had difficulty discussing some of the issues, especially when talking about the split from her ex-partner. In the actor's brief it clearly states that this is a difficult subject for her and therefore she may have been reluctant to tell you everything. She may have paused mid-sentence or perhaps shown you that she was unsure as to whether to continue. You should have actively encouraged her at these points showing sympathy and empathy, e.g.

- *'I can understand this is a sensitive subject to discuss. Take your time.'*
- *'Please go on.'*
- *'Oh dear! Tell me a little more about what happened.'*

4. **Respond to cues that lead to a deeper understanding of the problem**
   In this scenario the patient/actor was told to come across quite anxious at first and then to give you clues later that she was quite down. You should have picked up on this. For example, she may not have revealed initially why she was worried, and when asked why she has come today she may have simply said, 'It's about Megan'. However, from her demeanour or her tone you may have felt that she was worried and wondered why. You may have replied:

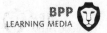

> *'You seem quite anxious today? Is everything alright?'*

Megan's mother may have then explained why she is anxious and the problems she is having with Megan.

It was also mentioned in the actor's brief that she is worried about a being a bad mother. Therefore, when you ask what she was hoping would happen today she may say:

> *'Well doctor. I think I need to get Megan sorted. I don't want to be accused of being a bad mother.'*

This would be a very big clue as she is talking about being 'accused'. Thus you may ask her:

> *'When you said that you didn't want to be accused of being a bad mother, what did you mean by that?'*

This may have then prompted her to reveal to you that her ex-partner is accusing her of being a bad mother or even her own feelings that she is a bad mother as she had an affair and caused Megan to be without her father.

5. **Elicit appropriate details to place the complaints in a social and psychosocial context**
    Although she has come about Megan there are clues from the brief that she may be having a few problems and may not be handling this whole situation well. First, she is concerned about her daughter, and second, she has recently split from her partner. These are difficult circumstances for anyone. Therefore it is vitally important to ask how this problem with Megan is affecting her.

> *   *'How is this problem with Megan affecting you?'*
> *   *'You mentioned that you have had a break-up with Megan's father. How are you coping with that?'*
> *   *'Do you have any friends and family you can confide in?'*

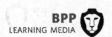

- *'Are you managing to cope financially now you are on your own?'*
- *'How are things between you and Megan's father after the break-up?'*

The patient may then respond to these questions by saying:

'To be honest I am not coping well. I am so worried about Megan that I am not sleeping or eating well. It is obviously difficult having broken up with Megan's father because we were together for many years and its difficult adjusting to being alone. The relationship between Megan's father and myself at the moment is rather strained. I do have friends and family around but I feel really embarrassed talking to them about what is going on . . . I think I might be a little depressed.'

The patient may then pause or stop there as she is reluctant to tell you more. She may need a little prompting especially as she says she feels embarrassed to talk about it. However, she has given you several clues to pick up on. If you miss the big clues such as her feeling too embarrassed to speak to her family and having a strained relationship with Megan's father, you may miss the underlying issues. Remember that everything the patient says is important. Therefore you may say:

- *'You mentioned you feel embarrassed. Why is that?'*
- *'I know you said you feel embarrassed discussing the situation but I would really like to find out more so that I can help you and Megan. Do you want to tell me a little more about what has happened?'*
- *'You mentioned that the relationship between you and Megan's father is strained. What did you mean by that?'*
- *'You mentioned that you think you may be depressed. What do you understand about depression?'*

This may encourage the patient to then reveal to you that she had an affair and feels guilty for putting Megan in this situation.

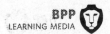

6. **Explore the patient's health understanding**

Here you need to explore the patient's ideas, concerns and expectations. This may include her beliefs around why Megan is behaving the way she is and her concerns regarding this, however it may also include her beliefs and concerns around her own mood. Therefore you may wish to ask.

- 'What is concerning you most about Megan's behaviour?'
- 'What are you worried will happen to Megan?'
- 'What do you think may be causing you to feel so low?'
- 'Is there anything you are worried that will happen if you continue to feel this way?'
- 'Have you any clues about why Megan may be acting this way?'
- 'Did you have any thoughts on what would happen today?'

This will allow the patient the chance to tell you that she thinks Megan's behaviour is due to the break-up with her partner and her worries surrounding this. She may also tell you that her low mood is due to her guilt around the situation and that she is worried she is depressed, if she had not told you this information already.

The patient may reply with:

- 'To be honest I don't think Megan is coping well with the split from her father. I'm worried as my parents broke-up when I was young and I didn't handle it well at all. I guess I'm worried that the same thing will happen to Megan. As I feel it is my fault that Megan's father left, as I'm the one that had the affair, I guess the guilt is getting me down. I think I may be depressed.'
- 'I'm worried that Megan's father will take her away from me. It is making me sick with worry.'

Once again you may need to do a little prompting picking up on the clues that she has given you.

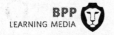

> • *'You mentioned that your parents broke-up when you were younger and that you did not handle it well at all. What did you mean by that?'*
> • *'You mentioned that you are worried that the same thing that happened to you as a child will happen to Megan. What did you mean by that?'*
> • *'You mentioned that you are worried Megan's father may take her away from you. What makes you think that?'*

This may be the extra encouragement she needs to tell you about her childhood and the fact that she ended up with the wrong crowd due to not talking to anyone about how she feels. She may also then tell you about Megan's father's threats to take her away as she is a 'bad mother'.

7. **Obtain sufficient information to include or exclude likely relevant significant conditions**
   In this scenario you really have two patients: Megan and her mother. You are told already that there are no child protection concerns and Megan is a completely healthy child. Therefore you do not need to take a full medical and developmental history surrounding Megan. However, you may need to ask her mother a bit more about what exactly Megan is doing that is concerning her, or if this is affecting her schooling, to give you a better idea of the situation. You may also wish to ask the mother a bit more about her mood and exclude any suicidal ideation as she has told you already that she is not coping.

> • *'How is Megan doing at school? Has this affected her academic achievements? Have you spoken to the school to see if Megan is having any problems there?'*
> • *'Is Megan eating and sleeping okay?'*
> • *'You mentioned earlier that you are not sleeping or eating well and feel you are not coping well. Have you had any thoughts of harming yourself?'*

The patient may then reply:

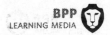

> *'Megan is absolutely fine with school and I don't want the school getting involved.'*

This abrupt response should raise alarms and you should obviously ask her why she seems so reluctant to have the school involved. She may then explain that she is worried that the school may contact her father or it may go on Megan's record and this give Megan's father the evidence that he needs to prove she is unfit as a mother.

Hopefully, if you have been sympathetic and listened to her mother she will open up to you about how she feels and her fears with getting anyone else involved.

8. **Choose an appropriate physical or mental examination**
   You will not need to do a physical examination in this case especially as Megan is not present. However, in real life you would probably be doing a mental state examination of her mother while she is talking to you. Here you may be assessing how she is dressed, if she has good eye contact with you or if she looks depressed. Therefore it is useful to do this during the mock consultation especially as it will give you a good idea of her mental state and allow you to pick up on any clues.

9. **Make a clinically appropriate working diagnosis / explain the diagnosis to the patient in appropriate language taking into account the patient's elicited beliefs**
   This case is ot about making a formal and official diagnosis as to what is causing Megan's behaviour problems, especially as she is not there for you to speak to her. However, her mother is there and as she has mentioned that she is not sleeping or eating and is feeling down it may be appropriate to explain to her that you agree that she may be depressed. It may also be appropriate to agree with her mother that it may be the break-up with her father that is causing Megan to be a little subdued. This shows that you are taking her beliefs into account when explaining to the patient what you feel is causing both her and Megan to feel so low. Again you will need to explain the situation in simple language so that the patient can understand.

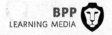

> *'I think you are right when you say that it may be the split from your ex that is causing Megan to be a little subdued. This is to be expected but I can understand why you are worried. You obviously have a lot of negative feelings towards yourself over what has happened and I think you are actually depressed. Do you understand what I mean by depression? (If the patient does not understand then explain what depression is.) What do you think?'*

10. **Make an appropriate management plan/involve the patient in significant management decisions**

    Your management plan may vary. You may decide to suggest that you refer Megan to a child psychologist or perhaps you may ask her to bring Megan in so you can assess the situation. With regards to Megan's mother you may offer her counselling or an anti-depressant. You may just offer her support and a friendly ear when she needs it. What decision you come to is not important however, you need to involve her in the decision making process.

    You may say something similar to this:

> *'Having discussed your concerns about Megan today there are various things we can do. One option would be to refer her to a specialist in this area who she could talk to. You mentioned earlier that you did not talk to anyone when something similar happened to you and therefore it may help Megan to have someone impartial she can speak to. On the other hand you could bring Megan to see me and we could have regular talks about how she is doing and keep an eye on things. What would you prefer?'*

This approach also takes into account her beliefs: i.e. that if Megan doesn't speak to someone it may get worse as it did for her. However, it also takes into account the fact that she is very worried about her ex-partner using anything against her and she may prefer you just keeping an eye on things. Therefore when you give her these options she may say:

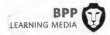

> '*I am really worried about Megan and I do think she needs someone to talk to. However, I am worried that if she sees a psychologist her father will find out and will use it to say I am a bad mother.*'

As her GP it is your job to do what is best for Megan. Therefore although it is her mother's decision as to whether she gets referred, you should make sure she does not make the decision to not refer her out of fear. Therefore you may need to say:

> '*I can understand why that would concern you. Many children find it difficult adjusting to their parents breaking up and I don't think anyone would view that as you being a bad mother. These things happen sometimes. The fact that you are here and trying to do something to help Megan is more than enough evidence that you care about her and are trying to do your best.*'

She should then be reassured and allow you to refer Megan to a child psychologist. However, had she not wanted this it would not have been appropriate to put pressure on her. Thankfully, in the brief the actor is told to allow you to refer her as long as you have been sympathetic and addressed her concerns.

When discussing your management plan for Megan's mother you may have suggested counselling or anti-depressants or even simply some time off work. Again the exact details of your plan are not important as long as you have given her the choice and allowed her to decide on what she feels is best for her.

11. **When prescribing take steps to enhance concordance by exploring and responding to the patient's understanding of the treatment**
    This would only be appropriate if you were going to prescribe an anti-depressant. However, as this case is quite lengthy and there are so many other issues, you may not have time to address how the anti-depressants work in detail. However, if you had some spare time you may have wanted to explain a little bit about them, for completeness sake, for example:

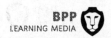

> - *'We have decided to start you on an anti-depressant. Do you know how these work?'*
> - *'Well they gradually increase the level of the happy chemical in the body. This will obviously not relieve all of your worries but it may help you to cope a little better with things. As it is a gradual process it may take four to six weeks for you to feel any better, so don't be disheartened if you don't feel an effect straight away.'*

12. **Specify the conditions and interval for follow up and review (safety net)**

    Again you may have different ideas for when she or Megan should be brought back. The important thing is to offer her some follow up and ensure you inform her that if things get bad or she has any thoughts of harming herself she should see you immediately. You will also need to ensure that if Megan deteriorates that you tell her to come back also, for example:

> *'I would like to see you in about two weeks' time to make sure that you are okay. Perhaps you may also want to book an appointment for Megan around that time so that I can see how she is doing as well. However, if you start to feel worse about yourself or have any thoughts of harming yourself please come and see me immediately. Also, if you feel that Megan's behaviour is worsening and she is becoming more withdrawn or you are concerned for her safety please see me or call me immediately.'*

13. **Confirm the patient's understanding**

    Here you need to take active steps to ensure the patient had understood. You may ask her to summarise what you have said or ask her what she has understood from your conversation today.

> *'We have said quite a lot today and I would like to make sure we are both clear about what we have decided to do to help you and Megan. Could you just summarise what we have agreed so I can ensure there is no confusion?'*

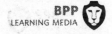

Again if you have explained everything appropriately the patient should understand and be happy with the diagnosis and plan. You can then simply ask if she has any more questions and end the consultation.

Notes

This case can be quite difficult if you do not pick up on the clues that the mother is giving you. Therefore you may have missed the fact that she was concerned that Megan would end up like her when she was that age or the fact that she was feeling quite guilty for the whole situation. If this happened to you then you need to ask yourself why that was. Perhaps you concentrated more on trying to solve the problem with Megan's behaviour and did not explore the mother's ideas, concerns and expectations? Or perhaps you didn't explore how Megan's behaviour was affecting her mother and how difficult it was for her to deal with this at this time. It may also be that you did not encourage her to continue speaking when she became reluctant or paused, as the actor was specifically told that she needed a lot of encouragement to reveal the information to you. If this was the case, try to replay the consultation, asking the necessary questions that you missed, and see if the consultation turns out differently.

The actor was also told to be reluctant to let you refer Megan to a child psychologist and for some of you, when Megan's mother refused to let you refer her you may have left it at that. Although you should respect her autonomy to decide what is best for her daughter, you cannot ignore the clues she has given you. Thus if she tells you that she is concerned about referring Megan, as Megan's father may use this against her, it would not be appropriate to simply ignore this and agree with her. You should at least try to explore this issue and reassure the mother that she is not a bad mother and is doing the right thing by arranging help for Megan. As stated before, had she still refused to let you refer Megan after this explanation, it would have been appropriate then to accept her wishes. However, at least you would have tried to reassure her and ensure she makes an informed decision and not one out of fear. In this scenario however, the actor was told to allow you to refer Megan if she felt sufficiently reassured. However, if she did not wish for you to refer Megan it is probably because you did not truly address her concerns or did not empathise enough with her situation.

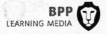

Mock Consultation 3

Doctor's brief

Mr Glen, a 45-year-old man, has come to see you for a sick certificate. He recently had a myocardial infarction four weeks ago but was told by the cardiac rehabilitation team that he should not go back to work for another two weeks. Therefore he has come to you to renew his sick certificate for another two weeks.

Additional information

Mr Glen is on the correct medication he needs to be after having a heart attack and is taking these correctly. Therefore there is no need to review his medication. He is no longer smoking. There is also no need to review his blood pressure, fasting glucose or cholesterol. These have been checked by the hospital and are all normal.

You have 10 minutes to complete this task.

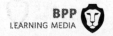

Use this space for your pre-consultation notes.

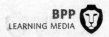

Mock Consultation 3

Patient's brief – *Do not read if you are playing the role of the doctor*

> Your name is Mr Glen and you are 45 years of age. You recently had a heart attack six weeks ago and need a sick certificate for the next two weeks. This is on the advice of the cardiac rehabilitation team who have told you not to go back to work until then.

Information unknown to the doctor

You have been suffering from tremendous anxiety since the heart attack. You worked as an investment banker and had a very stressful job before you became unwell. This heart attack came as a complete shock to you as you have always been healthy all your life. You are therefore convinced that it is the stress from your job that caused the heart attack. As such, you are quite worried about going back to work in case it triggers off another heart attack again.

You are not sleeping well due to your worries and are very anxious to do anything around the house in case you over-exert yourself. Although you have been told that it is perfectly safe to resume sexual intercourse, you are worried that this too may precipitate another heart attack. As a result it is affecting your relationship with your wife and this is also concerning you.

Your fears are worsened by the fact that your father died of a heart attack at 52 and you are worried that the same thing will happen to you if you are not careful.

Initially, when you come in, you reveal little as to what you are really worried about and simply ask the doctor for another certificate. You come across as unconcerned about your heart attack and give little clues that the experience has frightened you quite deeply. However, if the doctor asks you specifically about how you feel about your heart attack and how you are coping, you reveal what you are concerned about and show the doctor that you are actually quite anxious.

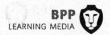

The issue regarding sex with your wife on the other hand is an embarrassing one and one you are not so eager to reveal. Therefore you will only tell the doctor about the sexual problems you are having if the doctor asks you about your relationship or home life in a sensitive manner and explores this more deeply.

You are also thinking about changing your job, due to your belief that it was the stress from your job that caused your heart attack. However, you do not reveal this to the doctor initially, and will only tell them if you feel that they have been sympathetic and have made you feel comfortable to reveal this information. As a result, if the doctor offers you various options to help you come to terms with your heart attack, you simply ask for some extra time off work to give you a chance to find another job. You think that you would like at least another month off to try and sort yourself out. If the doctor has not explored your concerns, however, you do not reveal to him anything about wishing to find a new job and simply take the sick note for another two weeks.

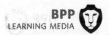

Mock Consultation 3

Information from brief

This brief is very short however there is some information that may be relevant.

Mr Glen, a 45-year-old man, has come to see you for a sick certificate

As we know already that the case in the assessment is unlikely to simply involve signing a sick certificate, therefore we need to keep an eye out for possible issues. The fact that the brief mentions his age may also be appropriate but we need to read on.

He recently had a myocardial infarction four weeks ago

He is obviously quite young to have a heart attack as he is only 45 years old. Why did this happen at such a young age? Did he have any heart problems previously? Did he have a strong family history of cardiac disease? Are there perhaps any modifiable risk factors that could have caused this e.g. cholesterol, smoking etc? However we are told in the brief that these are all normal and he has already stopped smoking. How has it affected him having a heart attack at such a young age? How is his family coping with this?

He was told by the cardiac rehabilitation team that he should not go back to work for another two weeks. Therefore he has come to you to renew his sick certificate

This seems pretty straightforward. However, if you are going to sign the certificate will you give it for just two weeks? Does he feel ready to go back to work then? There is obviously some underlying issue in this case as it seems too straightforward.

Additional information

This is telling you that medically there is no need to review the patient today as his fasting glucose, cholesterol and blood pressure are all fine and he is on the correct medication. Therefore you do not need to waste time taking a history or reviewing these risk factors as this has already been addressed. As you are told that he has given up smoking there is no need to go into this either.

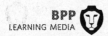

Mock Consultation 3

Suggested approach to the consultation by the doctor

1. **Creating a safe environment for the patient**

   Here you need to ensure that the furniture is carefully arranged as you would for any consultation. As you should have been suspicious that there was a hidden agenda, you should have ensured that you were suitably placed to watch the patient's expressions and manners to pick up on any non-verbal clues. You should however, have not been too close to the patient that it became uncomfortable, and therefore the patient should not have needed to adjust his position once the consultation had started.

   Again you should have maintained eye contact throughout the consultation, to reassure the patient that you were listening, as well as to pick up on any non-verbal clues. You should have also paid attention to your body language and your tone, making sure that you showed the patient you were interested in what they had to say and that you were sympathetic to how they were feeling.

2. **Introduction and opening statement**

   You should have greeted the patient and invited him in. As you were given the patient's name in the brief you should have used it. There is no mention as to whether you knew the patient or not beforehand, so as a precaution you should have introduced yourself. It may be that the patient then tells you that perhaps he has seen you once before, but as you are not given that information it is perfectly acceptable to introduce who you are.

   Although the brief says that the patient is coming to renew his sick certificate, you should have still used an open question for your opening statement. This would allow the patient to perhaps give you some extra clues as to whether there may be something else going on. As you are suspecting that there may be an underlying issue, you should be paying close attention to the patient during their response.

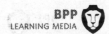

Examples of an appropriate introduction and opening statement would be:

- *'Hello Mr Glen, please come in. I don't believe we have met before, have we? Oh, I didn't think so. I'm Doctor W, how can I help you today?'*
- *'Hello Mr Glen, please have a seat. I'm Doctor W. Pleased to meet you. Would you like to tell me what has brought you here today?'*

3. **Encourage the patient's contribution at appropriate points in the consultation**

As the patient has come to you with a hidden agenda, you should have needed to encourage them to tell you more, to be able to get to the root of the problem. The actor was told not to reveal initially what he was concerned about and to simply come across as if he wanted a sick certificate. He may have simply said, 'I just need another sick note doctor' when you asked him what had brought him to see you today.

Therefore you would have needed to encourage the patient to go on and you might have said:

- *'Oh, you have been unwell recently?' (Pausing to let the patient continue and tell you what has happened with regards to his heart attack.)*
- *'Oh dear, you have been off work? What happened?'*

This should have hopefully allowed him the opportunity to tell you about his heart attack allowing you to pick up on other clues. Obviously, there may have been other points later in the consultation where he became hesitant or perhaps paused prematurely. Again, you would have needed to encourage him to continue perhaps by saying:

- *'Please tell me more.'*
- *'Oh dear, that must have been awful. Please continue.'*

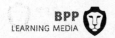

You should have also showed that you were listening to the patient, therefore encouraging him to continue his story, by nodding your head or perhaps making simple verbal gestures such as 'hmm' during the time he was talking. This may sound silly but it is important for the patient to know that you are interested and paying attention to what he is saying.

4. **Respond to cues that lead to a deeper understanding of the problem**

In this scenario the patient/actor was told specifically to not initially reveal his concerns. Therefore it was up to you to pick up on the clues that perhaps there was something else going on. As the actor was told to show little in his mannerisms, there may have been other signs to indicate something was wrong. For example, had he responded to your comment of 'oh, have you been unwell recently?' He may have replied:

> *'Oh yes, doctor. I was in hospital. It was nothing serious, I just had a heart attack but I'm okay now.'*

This should immediately have made you wonder what the patient meant. He says he 'just had a heart attack'. Surely being in hospital and having a heart attack at 45 years of age would be a frightening experience for anyone? Therefore it may be that he is genuinely not concerned over what has happened, but it may be that he is covering up his feelings. Therefore, you need to respond yet again to this clue and explore it in more detail. You may ask:

> *'A heart attack? That must have been frightening for you, especially at your age? You must have been very shocked when this happened.'*

As you have now shown some insight and empathy into how the patient feels, he may now feel comfortable to tell you that it indeed was a shock:

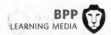

> *'Well, doctor, I guess it was a bit of a shock as I've always been healthy. I mean it's not normal for young men like me to have a heart attack, is it? But then again, that's life, isn't it? Anything can happen.'*

Obviously this statement is full of clues for you to pick up on, as the patient has given you an insight into his health beliefs. This is then an excellent opportunity to discuss his ideas, concerns and expectations later based on this statement.

5. **Elicit appropriate details to place the complaints in a social and psychosocial context**
   From the brief we have already contemplated the idea that as a relatively young man, having a heart attack may have had a significant impact on his life. Therefore it is important to ask about the psychological, social and financial aspects it may have had on his life. Consequently you may have asked:

> - *'How has the heart attack affected you?'*
> - *'What has this whole experience stopped you from doing?'*
> - *'Obviously you are meant to be taking it easy at this time. How are you coping with that?'*
> - *'How has this affected your family? They must have also been very shocked that this has happened to you?'*
> - *'How have your employers been with regards to you taking time off? Have they been supportive?'*
> - *'How do you feel about taking time off work?'*

This may prompt the patient to reveal a little more information than they anticipated; especially if they were just expecting for you to sign the sick note. The patient may respond with something like this:

> *'Well, obviously I am a little nervous to do too much as I have been told to take it easy. I have always been a really busy person so it's not easy to just sit around and do nothing. Work has been okay about me taking time off. I mean they should be, it's their fault I'm in this situation in the first place. As for the family, well obviously they are worried. It's not easy on my wife you know ... having a man in this condition ...'*

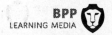

The patient has given you numerous clues in this statement. However the ones that really stand out are about work being the reason he is in this predicament and also when he mentions that it is not easy having a man in 'this condition'. Therefore, you should try to clarify this and gain a deeper insight into what the patient means.

- *'You mentioned that it is not easy for your wife having a man in this condition. What did you mean by that?'*
- *'When you said that it is work's fault for you being in this predicament could you tell me a little more about what you meant?'*

This is obviously trying to find out what the patient understands about his health and the implications.

6. Explore the patient's health understanding

We have already just mentioned a few statements you could use to address this criteria, mostly involving exploring what the patient means about work putting him in this predicament, as this could assist our understanding of what the patient believes caused his heart attack. Earlier on we also had an example of another clue mentioned by the patient, that we could pick up on and explore to try and find out what the patient understands about his health and what his concerns are. This was the clue the patient gave us when he mentioned that it was not normal for a young healthy man to have a heart attack.

'Well, doctor, I guess it was a bit of a shock as I've always been healthy. I mean it's not normal for young men like me to have a heart attack is it? But then again that's life isn't it? Anything can happen.'

There you may have wanted to pick up on this and reflected it back to the patient saying:

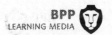

> *'Earlier on you mentioned that you did not think it was normal for men your age to have a heart attack. What did you mean by this? Have you had any thoughts on what may have caused this to happen to you?'*

This may then lead on to the patient telling you that he has had a very stressful job which he thinks caused this problem. He may have also told you this when you asked what he meant when he said that work had put him in this predicament. This is just another way of eliciting the same information.

You should then have gone on to explore the patient's concerns and expectations, now that you understood what he felt had caused the heart attack. Earlier on we mentioned that the patient may have implied that there was a problem between him and his wife, when he mentioned that it was not easy for his wife having a man in 'this condition'. We decided that we should reflect this back to the patient and explore this by asking him what he meant by this comment. The patient may have then gone on to say:

> *'Well, doctor, obviously it will be a very long time till I can have sex again and that is not going to be easy on our relationship.'*

This again is a health belief and is a false one. This would then have given you an opportunity to discuss why the patient feels that way and if this is his belief or something he has been told. If you address this the patient should hopefully tell you that although he has been told he can resume sexual intercourse, he is worried to do so in case he has another heart attack. Therefore, you have now started to address some of the patient's concerns.

To explore the patient's concerns in more detail you may want to ask him directly what he is worried about or what his concerns for his future are:

> *'What is concerning you the most over what has happened to you? What do you expect to happen in the future?'*

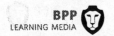

This may prompt the patient to tell you that he is extremely worried about having another heart attack particularly as his father died of a heart attack at the age of 52. He may also reveal to you that he is worried about going back to work, as he feels this may trigger off another heart attack, and that he expects if he continues in his current job that this is what will happen. He may also tell you that because of this he is seriously considering changing job. If you have revealed all this information, you have now fully explored his ideas, concerns and expectations and now have a much deeper understanding of the case.

7. **Obtain sufficient information to include or exclude likely relevant significant conditions**
In this case you are specifically told that his risk factors for heart disease, e.g. blood pressure, cholesterol and diabetes have already been checked at the hospital and are all normal. Therefore you do not need to take a full medical clerking as you would if a patient presented with acute chest pain. As he has just had a heart attack, however, it may be appropriate to ask him if he is feeling well and if he has had any chest pains. This is because if he has had any chest pains it may be significant and you may need to refer him back to the hospital urgently.

Some of you may have felt it appropriate to ask him if he started smoking again, as if he had started smoking you may be able to offer him further support to quit. You may have also asked him about his lifestyle before the heart attack to see if his diet and exercise regime could be improved. Although this is perfectly acceptable and good practice, however you would not have gained many marks for this. This is because this case is more about eliciting the patient's worries and not about the medical management of a heart disease patient. Therefore if you addressed this it should have been done briefly and promptly.

Depending on how the case went some of you may have also felt it appropriate to check for biological features of depression, e.g. early morning waking, anhedonia, lack of appetite. For some of you the patient would have given you no concerns

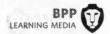

that he was suffering from depression and thus if you did not ask for these do not worry. The actor's brief said nothing about the patient being depressed so these questions were not necessary.

8. **Choose an appropriate physical or mental examination**
As we have stated numerous times you are unlikely to have to do an examination in the assessment. However, we did mention that it may be appropriate sometimes to mention that you will examine the patient after your discussion. Therefore although you would not gain many extra marks for this, you may have mentioned to the patient that you will listen to their heart and check their blood pressure after your discussion to make sure everything is okay. This would give the patient extra reassurance and thus you may have felt it necessary to mention this as the patient was worried. If you had not mentioned this however, it would have made little difference to your overall mark.

9. **Make a clinically appropriate working diagnosis / explain the diagnosis to the patient in appropriate language taking into account the patient's elicited beliefs**
This case does not involve making a formal diagnosis. We already know the patient has got ischaemic heart disease. It is more perhaps explaining to the patient what a heart attack could be caused by and what he can expect in the future. The patient should have told us several of their health beliefs during the consultation, and these should be mentioned in our explanation to the patient. Therefore, some useful explanations of what has happened to the patient may involve the following:

- *'Mr Glen it has obviously come as a shock to you that a fit healthy man like yourself has had a heart attack. This is even of greater concern when your father died of a heart attack at a young age, and it is natural that you would be worried about the same thing happening to you.'*
- *'You are right in saying that this it is unusual for a young person like yourself, who has always been healthy to have a heart attack. There are several things that can increase*

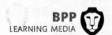

your risk of having a heart attack. One of these is smoking, and thankfully you have now given this up, but this may have been a major contributing factor to what happened to you.'

- 'Having someone in the family who has had heart problems is also a big risk factor for having a heart attack. Therefore the fact that your father had a heart attack at a very young age may have put you at increased risk of having a heart attack at a similarly young age. Obviously, emotional stress can bring on a heart attack, but it more usual for this to happen to people who already have other reasons to have a heart problem. Therefore it is unlikely that it was your job alone that caused the heart attack. It is likely to be a combination of factors, these factors being your family history of heart disease and your smoking. Does that make sense?'

- 'You have mentioned that you are concerned to have sexual intercourse with your wife and that you are concerned to go back to work in case you have another heart attack. Although we cannot change your family history and you are naturally concerned about your heart in view of what happened to your father, there is no reason that you cannot go back to enjoying the things you used to. The cardiac rehabilitation team is completely correct; you can safely resume sexual intercourse with your wife. Normal sexual activity is no more strenuous on the heart than a number of normal physical activities such as brisk walking or carrying some shopping, so there really is no cause for concern.'

- 'Also as I have said previously, it is unlikely that it was the stress of your job alone that caused this heart attack, although it may not have helped matters. Obviously, you know more than I do, as to how stressful your job is and whether there is any way the stress can be avoided. However, we do have you on a lot of different tablets, and this coupled with the fact you have give up smoking, means that we have dramatically lowered the chances of this happening to you again. Therefore I think it is unlikely that a simple stressful situation would put you at any significant risk of having another heart attack. However, I can fully appreciate why after such a major event you would be keen to avoid any unnecessary worries.'

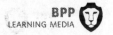

The patient may then tell you that he feels more reassured, however he still feels it would be in his best interest to look for another job. This is entirely his decision and at least he is now making an informed decision, realising that it is unlikely that it was his job alone that caused his heart attack.

10. **Make an appropriate management plan/involve the patient in significant management decisions**

Your management plan may vary depending on how the case went and you may offer the patient a variety of alternatives. Obviously the patient has come to you for a sick note, and does not feel ready to go back to work, so this should be part of your management plan. However, you may have offered some other suggestions such as counselling or the names and numbers of support groups for the patient.

> * *'Mr Glen, you are obviously not physically or mentally ready to go back to work as yet. Would you agree with that? I am quite happy to give you another sick note in view of this. You mentioned you would like two weeks off? Do you think this would be enough time? I could give you slightly longer if you like or we could give you two weeks and see how you are feeling then. If you need more time off at that point we could extend your sick note. What would you prefer?'*
> * *'Mr Glen, understandably having such a major thing happen to you has affected you quite deeply. Have you thought about maybe speaking to someone about how this has made you feel? For example, we could refer you for counselling on a one to one basis, or perhaps I could give you the contact of some support groups. That way you could talk to other people who have been through a similar experience to you which may help you. What do you think?'*

The patient should then mention that he would just like some more time off work to try and get better and also to find another job. Therefore, you may have agreed to give him four weeks off work, which he should have asked you for if the consultation had gone to plan.

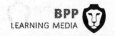

11. **When prescribing take steps to enhance concordance by exploring and responding to the patient's understanding of the treatment**
    As you are not prescribing anything in this circumstance this point is not relevant.

12. **Specify the conditions and interval for follow up and review (safety net)**
    The exact details of what follow up you have given may have varied. However, if you had issued the sick note for four weeks as the patient requested, you should have told the patient to come back if he still feels unready to go back to work at that time. You should have also mentioned to the patient that if he has any chest pains he should seek medical attention straight away, as this is vitally important.

13. **Confirm the patient's understanding**
    You should have taken steps to ensure that the patient has understood what you had said. As a result, you may have asked him to summarise what had been said today. Therefore you may have said something like this to the patient:

> • *'If you were to go home and perhaps tell your wife what we have discussed today. What would you say?'*
> • *'Just so I can ensure we are both clear would you like to tell me the main points that we have discussed today?'*

This should lead on to the patient clearly summarising what you have discussed and is an excellent way to end the consultation. It is always good practice to ask the patient at the end if they have any further questions. As long as you have explained everything correctly the patient should say 'no'. However, if something was not clear they may ask you to explain this again. Although this is not ideal it is far better than the patient going home confused.

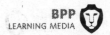

Notes

This consultation is an excellent example of a patient's hidden agenda, and how asking the correct questions can reveal a lot of hidden information from what seemed a straightforward case. As chest pain is a medical problem, and one that all of you should feel quite comfortable dealing with, you may have spent too long exploring the medical aspect of the presenting complaint. Therefore you may have gone to great lengths to ensure that he was medically fit, and wanted to examine the patient asking him whether he was suffering from any chest pains, palpitations or shortness of breath. Although it is important to ensure that he is well and has not had any further chest pains, this can be quickly excluded by the use of two simple closed questions. Therefore, it was not appropriate to go into great lengths about his chest pain and his current symptoms.

Although the patient was anxious about having another heart attack, he was worried mostly about his work and sexual intercourse bringing this on. He was not worried that his cholesterol was high or that his blood pressure may be abnormal. Therefore, although it is generally appropriate to discuss modifiable risk factors in these patients to try and reduce the risk of a further heart attack, this would not have addressed *this* patient's concerns. Therefore, if you went to great lengths to reassure the patient that he should be fine as he is on the correct medications, has normal bloods and blood pressure and is now an ex-smoker, you were unlikely to have made him feel any better. You needed to have specifically addressed his concerns about going back to work and having sex with his wife.

If you did not elicit these concerns, replay the consultation spending more time exploring the psychosocial aspect of his presenting complaint as well as his ideas, concerns and expectations. If you get stuck, try using some of the phrases we have used in the suggested approach, or ask your colleagues for suggestions.

Finally, if you ended up simply signing the sick certificate for another two weeks and not for the four weeks that the patient actually wanted, try to figure out why this was. Perhaps you missed the issues completely and just took what he said on face value, believing he just wanted another two weeks off work?

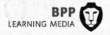

Or perhaps you were not sympathetic enough for the patient to reveal to you his concerns over his job and the fact that he needed more time before returning to work. Once again, if this was the case simply replay the consultation from where it went wrong, using some of the example phrases we have suggested to see if the outcome is any different.

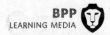

Mock Consultation 4

Doctor's brief

You are a doctor working on a colorectal surgical team. Mrs Patel, a 60-year-old lady, has come to see you for her colonoscopy and biopsy results. She was referred by her GP for a colonoscopy as she had rectal bleeding and a change in bowel habit. Unfortunately, the colonoscopy and biopsy results confirm that she has bowel cancer. She had been previously seen by your Consultant, Miss Brown, and her Registrar, Mr Green, before, however you have been asked to see her today. You have never met her before.

Additional information

The biopsy results are certain that this is cancer. The patient has not had any further tests such as a CT scan so you are unsure about the staging of the cancer and therefore the prognosis at this stage. She will need to have a CT scan of her chest, abdomen and pelvis as well as another appointment after that to discuss the results.

You have 10 minutes to complete this task.

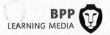

Use this space for your pre-consultation notes.

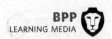

Mock Consultation 4

Patient's brief – *Do not read if you are playing the role of the doctor*

> You are Mrs Patel a 60-year-old lady who had seen your GP with rectal bleeding and a change in bowel habit. He referred you for a colonoscopy which you had at the hospital as well as a biopsy. You have come back today for the results. You were last seen by the Consultant Miss Brown and her Registrar Mr Green. You have never seen the doctor you are seeing today before.

Information unknown to the doctor

You have come alone today as your husband has travelled to India and will be there for the next couple of months. You are meant to fly out next week to meet him. You are not worried about the result of the colonoscopy, as you think the bleeding is probably caused by piles, and have no idea it could be cancer. Your husband felt the same way as he too had rectal bleeding and had the same tests. In the end he was told it was simple piles, and therefore both you and he are convinced that you have the same problem. You had only gone to the GP to collect a prescription for some haemorrhoid cream that your husband used, but the GP referred you for this test. He did not really explain why he was referring you and therefore you are not expecting anything sinister.

You are very keen to know the results so you can put this behind you and join your husband. Therefore at first you are quite eager to hear the results. If the doctor asks you how much you want to know about the results, you initially ask them to 'tell you what you need to know'. The doctor will then inform you that it is cancer. This will come as major shock to you and you react quite badly, becoming very emotional and upset. You are not prepared to deal with this today, especially when you are alone. You will be in denial about the situation and ask the doctor several questions about how they are so sure it is cancer. You were unaware that a biopsy was taken, and you only accept the diagnosis if the doctor explains what the biopsy is and therefore how they can be certain this is cancer.

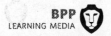

Once you have been told the bad news, you do not want to know the in depth details about the cancer, and what treatments you may need to have. If the doctor begins to go into any details about surgery or chemotherapy you become even more upset. However, if the doctor asks you how much more you wish to know in advance, you simply ask him if it can be cured. You also tell him that you would prefer to come back with a relative before he gives you all the details. The doctor should tell you that they cannot answer whether your cancer is curable until they know how advanced the cancer is and if it has spread. They may also tell you that you need to have a scan to find this out.

You want your husband with you and will only agree to come back once he returns from India. However, you not think he will return for at least another two to three weeks. You do not seem to understand the importance of having the scan as soon as possible and are insistent that you cannot do anything until your husband is with you. This is because you do not want to make any decisions without him and usually always make decisions with his input. However if the doctor is sympathetic to how you feel, and explains that you will not need to make any decisions at the scan appointment, you agree to bring another relative with you if your husband is not back in time. You would still prefer to wait until the follow up appointment after the scan to hear all the details as you are certain that your husband will be back by then.

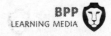

Mock Consultation 4

Information from brief

Things you may have picked up from the brief are:

Mrs Patel, a 60-year-old lady, has come to see you for her colonoscopy and biopsy results

The name Patel would imply that she is of Asian origin or perhaps married into an Asian family. Although it may have no relevance at all it may be important to take this into account especially when trying to understand her beliefs.

She was referred by her GP for a colonoscopy as she had rectal bleeding and a change in bowel habit

These symptoms are obviously worrying. As she has been referred by her GP you are unsure as to what she has been told by the GP. This may be important to find out as you need to know whether she was warned about the possibility of this being anything serious.

Unfortunately, the colonoscopy and biopsy results confirm that she has bowel cancer

Therefore you are aware that this is a situation where you will have to break bad news. As a result you need to think about what the important factors are when breaking bad news and be prepared for the patient to exhibit a wide range of emotions.

She had been previously seen by your Consultant, Miss Brown, and her Registrar, Mr Green, before however, you have been asked to see her today. You have never met her before

As the patient has never met you before it may be difficult to break bad news to her. You may feel uncomfortable in this situation and should ensure that your discomfort is not apparent to the patient during this sensitive time. Also you will have absolutely no clue what she has been told by the rest of your team, as you were not there at the time, so again it will be important to find out what she knows already.

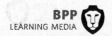

139

The biopsy results are certain that this is cancer

Why are you being told this? Is there a possibility that the patient may think that there has been a mistake made? However, you are told specifically by this statement that this is not the case. The diagnosis is clear.

The patient has not had any further tests such as a CT scan so you are unsure about the staging of the cancer and therefore the prognosis at this stage

This is giving you an indication that you are in no position to talk about prognosis with this patient so that there is probably no need to do this in the consultation.

She will need to have a CT scan of her chest, abdomen and pelvis as well as another appointment after that to discuss the results

This is telling you what should be included in your management plan and therefore you are likely to need to mention this at some point.

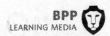

Mock Consultation 4

Suggested approach to the consultation by the doctor

1. **Setting up**

   You should have been aware that this would be a difficult consultation. You are about to tell someone they have cancer, and you should have been prepared to experience a wide variety of emotions from the patient. Therefore the room should have been set up appropriately. There should not have been any furniture or obstacles between you and the patient that could have blocked your view or broken eye contact. You should have also ensured that your chair was placed at an appropriate angle, where you could see the patient's facial expressions at all times, and pick up on any non-verbal clues. It was also important to have placed your chair close enough to the patient to have been able to reach out and offer a comforting hand if they became upset. If there were tissues in the room, these should have been placed at an arm's length away or less from both you and the patient, so that they were easily accessible.

   Obviously in real life you would have ensured that the door was closed and that there were no interruptions. This is likely to be irrelevant for the assessment as there are unlikely to be any phones or interruptions in the assessment.

   You should have invited the patient in calling her by her name as it was given to you in the brief. There is a specific comment informing you that you have never met Mrs Patel before. Therefore you should have introduced who you were. It may have also been useful to explain that you are still part of the same team of doctors that Mrs Patel had seen before.

   > *'Mrs Patel, good morning, please come in and have a seat. I believe you saw Miss Brown the Consultant and her Registrar Mr Green the last time you were here? My name is Dr Crystal, I am another one of the doctors working for Miss Brown on the team, pleased to meet you.'*

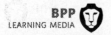

The brief states that Mrs Patel is coming alone. Obviously as you know you are going to give her bad news this is not ideal. You should ideally have offered her the opportunity to have a friend or relative present. This needed to be done tactfully as you obviously did not want to indicate to the patient that there was bad news before you have had a chance to explain. You may have wished to say something like this:

> *'Have you come alone today, Mrs Patel? Would you prefer to have someone with you?'*

The patient may then have told you that she would have preferred someone to be with her, but her husband is abroad in India at the moment. You may then have needed to ask her how long he was away for, to see if it was feasible to wait for him to be present to break the news. She may have then told you that he wouldn't be back for three months, so that she is fine by herself today, as she just wants to know the results.

As the actor's brief states that she is not suspecting anything wrong, and is keen to know the results, she may have simply told you that does not need anyone with her. In either case she clearly gives you the impression that she is quite happy for you to give her the results here and now.

2. **Perception**
You should have taken active steps to find out what the patient understood already. This involves finding out if she understood why she had the colonoscopy and also what she thinks it found. Therefore you may have asked:

> *'Mrs Patel, we have asked you to come back today to give you the results of the camera test that you had last week. Do you understand why you had this test?'*

The patient, who was told in the brief that she did not really understand why she had the colonoscopy, may respond with:

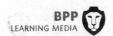

> *'Well, I am not really sure. I think it was to find out if I had piles. I was bleeding from the back passage and my motions were loose so I went to see my doctor because I thought I had piles. My husband uses this cream for the same problem as he has bleeding from the back passage too. I just wanted the doctor to prescribe me some of the cream my husband uses. The next thing I know I'm being told I need a camera test up the back passage.'*

This has told you that Mrs Patel may not be expecting bad news at all. It seems like she feels she just has simple haemorrhoids, and it does not appear that the GP explained why they were referring her for this test. However, it is best not to assume, so you should have taken active steps to find out what her GP has told her or explained to her about what the test could find.

> *'Did your GP explain what we might be looking for when we do this test?'*

The patient should then tell you that the GP did not explain what a colonoscopy could find, as stated in the actor's brief. However, in other cases you may find that the GP did explain that they may find something abnormal, but the patient is in denial and does not mention this.

> *'No, Dr Crystal, he didn't. But my husband had the same test, when he also had bleeding from the back passage, and he was told he had piles. So I'm assuming it's to check for the same thing?'*

You should have now been certain that Mrs Patel is convinced that she has piles, and was not informed that the reason she was going to have a colonoscopy, was to exclude any other serious conditions. At this point, you should have explained to the patient why she was referred for a colonoscopy, and what a colonoscopy could find. This would have allowed you to gently lead into breaking the bad news to the patient.

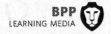

> *'Mrs Patel, you are correct in saying that bleeding from the back passage can be caused by piles. However, it does not normally cause you to have loose motions that you described. Because of this, your doctor felt it necessary to try to find out what was causing both the bleeding and the loose motions. One of the best ways to do that is to put a camera into the back passage and to have a look at the bowel. This can tell us if there is problem with the bowel, such as infection, and can also tell us if there are any growths in the bowel which can also cause these symptoms. If we do see an area that looks abnormal we can also take a small sample from the area. This is called a biopsy. We can then examine this area in more detail under a microscope to find out if there is anything to worry about. Does this all make sense?'*

3. Invitation

Now that you should have explained to the patient what a colonoscopy is, and what it may have been used for, you should have taken active steps to find out exactly how much the patient wanted to know about the test results. At least now the patient should have a slight idea that it is possible that her symptoms could have been caused by something abnormal.

> *'Last week when you came to see us we did the camera test to see if we could find out what was causing your symptoms. We did see an area of your bowel that looked different from the rest of the bowel and we did a biopsy of that area. The results of both the camera test and the biopsy results are now back. How much about these results would you like to know?'*

The actor was told to not be worried initially and so should have been quite happy for you to tell her the results. Thus the patient may have replied along these lines:

> *'Well, doctor, tell me what I should know. I'm sure everything is fine.'*

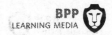

4. **Knowledge**

The patient told you that she wanted you to tell her what she 'should know'. This is obviously not very specific. However, she does need to know that she has cancer. Therefore, you should not delay any further and explained the results to her.

> '*Mrs Patel, unfortunately the tests have shown that you have cancer.*'

You should have paused here to allow the patient to take this in. It is more appropriate to just use the word cancer at this stage instead of bowel cancer as most patients will only hear the word 'cancer'. You should not have made this statement complicated or given any explanation of the type of cancer, prognosis or anything else. The patient needed to be able to absorb this information. You should also have made the diagnosis quite clear. Most patients understand the word 'cancer'. However terms like malignancy or neoplasm can be confusing to a patient and you should have avoided using any of this jargon. You should have also avoided saying anything ambiguous such as 'we have found something abnormal'. You needed to be clear.

The patient may then have asked you questions after this or perhaps was in shock and did not say anything. Again, you needed to have asked the patient for her permission to continue or give her any more information. Therefore you may have said:

> '*I understand this is a big shock for you. Would you like me to continue or do you need a little time?*'

The patient at this point could have reacted in a number of ways. They may have burst into tears or became angry. They may have simply asked you to continue. The actor's brief states that the patient became very upset and emotional and you should have allowed the patient time and space to vent their feelings. The actor was also told that she should also be in denial and not accept the diagnosis.

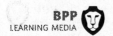

> *'Doctor, I don't understand this at all. Are you sure I don't have piles? How could this be happening? You must have got it wrong. I am sure it is just piles.'*

Although it is always possible that a mistake has been made, it was not appropriate to give the patient false hope about this. Therefore, although you needed to be understanding and sympathetic, you also needed to be quite clear about the diagnosis.

> *'Mrs Patel, I can completely appreciate that you were not expecting this, especially when your husband had the same test and was told he simply had piles. It must be very difficult for you to accept this and you must be wondering why this has happened to you. I am afraid that the sample we have taken from the bowel wall, the biopsy, is conclusive. We have examined it in great detail and unfortunately it is cancer. There is no mistake.'*

The patient may then have replied with:

> *'Oh, you took a biopsy. Okay. So it is cancer. Okay.'*

You should have again paused after giving the patient this information so that they could take it in and process it. You should have not rushed the patient or tried to give them any more information too soon. However, once you had allowed the patient time to come to terms with the diagnosis, you should have found out how much more she wanted to know.

> *'Earlier you said to me that you would like to know everything you need to know. Do you still feel that way? Would you like to know what will happen now?'*

The actor was specifically told to tell you that they do not want you to give them any more details until their husband is here. However, the actor should have asked you whether their cancer can be cured.

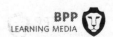

> *'Doctor, I don't think you should tell me anything until my husband is here. I want him to be here with me when you explain. I don't want to know any more please. All I want to know is can I be cured? Can I be cured, doctor?'*

This is obviously a very difficult question and you needed to be sensitive in your response. Your brief stated that you had no clue as to how advanced the cancer was and that the patient needed to have a CT scan to find this out. However, the patient has clearly told you that she is not ready for the finer details. Therefore you needed to be honest but to have given a very superficial response:

> *'I can understand why you would want your husband here at this time, and I am quite happy to explain everything to both you and him once he is back. Until we know a little more about the cancer it is difficult to tell you whether you can be cured. We will need to do a scan of your body to find out how big the cancer is, and if it has stayed in the bowel, before we can answer these questions. How do you feel about this?'*

The patient who has been told to be reluctant to do anything without her husband may have said:

> *'Okay, doctor, so I will need a scan? I don't want to have the scan without my husband present. Can it wait until he's back?'*

Obviously you should have enquired, if you had not found out already, when her husband would be back. The actor should have told you that her husband may not be back for another three to four weeks. Obviously this may have a significant impact on her prognosis and care and therefore you should have explained this to the patient. If she had still decided to wait for her husband you would have had to respect that, but at least she would be making an informed decision. You should have also tried to find out why she feels that she cannot have the scan until her husband is there. Is it because she is scared and wants support? Or is it because she does not feel comfortable making any decisions without involving him?

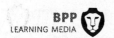

> *'I can understand this must be very frightening for you Mrs Patel, and very hard on you, especially as your husband is abroad. What is concerning you most however about having the scan when your husband is not here?'*

The patient should then have explained to you what was on the actor's brief, which is that she did not want to make any decisions without her husband. You should have responded to this is in a sensitive and non-judgemental manner.

> *'I can completely understand why you want your husband here and are not comfortable making any decisions without him. We could wait until he comes back to have the scan if you wish. However, it is important to have the scan as soon as possible. This way we can form a better picture of what we are dealing with and it will help us decide how we can help you. You will not need to make any decisions on the day you have your scan. You will simply come and go into a machine like a tunnel to have the scan. The whole appointment should not take much longer than thirty minutes and you will be able to go home afterwards.'*

This is quite a lot of information so it is useful to pause here to let the patient take in what you have said.

> *'We would then arrange a follow-up appointment to explain the results to you and it is likely that by this time your husband would be back. You could therefore bring him to this appointment. How do you feel about that?'*

The patient should then have agreed to come for the scan, saying that she would bring another relative with her for the appointment.

5. **Emotions**

We have already discussed a wide range of emotions that the patient may have expressed in this consultation. Initially, the actor should have been extremely upset and emotional when told she has cancer. You should have allowed her this time to express how she feels and should not have tried to interrupt

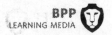

her. You should have remained quiet at this point and may have offered her a tissue or placed a hand on her shoulder for support. Once you have given her a little time to come to terms with this you may have empathised with the patient saying things such as:

> - *'I know this must be difficult for you.'*
> - *'I can understand this news is very upsetting.'*
> - *'I know this must have come as a shock to you.'*

The actor was then told to go into a stage of denial where she is not accepting of the diagnosis. This is a common reaction. You should again have listened to how the patient felt as well as showed that you understood why the patient felt that way. You have already gathered that the patient was not expecting this news at all and this would explain why it would be difficult for her to accept this diagnosis.

> *'I can understand this is difficult for you to accept. Especially when you were not expecting bad news.'*

As stated previously, although you should be sympathetic to the patient who is going through a phase of denial, you do need to make sure they understand there is no mistake. It would be harmful to the patient to give them any idea that perhaps the results were wrong as this would be giving them false hope. You do not need to go into great detail on the issue again. You should simply tell them that there is no mistake and that they do have cancer.

6. **Strategy and Summary**
    If you have been sympathetic and explained everything properly, the patient should have agreed to come in for the scan without her husband. Therefore your strategy should have been along the lines of offering the patient an appointment for the scan and explaining that she would have a follow up appointment after that. The patient clearly stated earlier that she did not want the details discussed without her husband, and thus the strategy should not have involved discussing possible treatments with her.

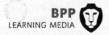

- 'Mrs Patel, I have explained to you that you need to come in to have a scan to tell us if the cancer has spread. Although, I completely understand that you would prefer if your husband was present, I have explained why I feel it is best for you to have this straight away. You have agreed to come for the scan with another one of your relatives and you will receive a letter in the post telling you when your appointment is. Is this okay?'
- 'After the scan you will receive another appointment to discuss the results of the scan and what will happen next. This will probably not be for another two to three weeks and therefore it is likely that your husband should be back by this time. If he is not back by then however, we could always postpone your appointment depending on how you feel. Would this be okay with you?'

Thus you have told the patient what to expect, and offered some sort of management plan, at the same time respecting her wishes that she prefers not to know too many details. Although, you may feel that this is a lot of detail already, you had no choice but to mention the scan as the patient asked you if she could be cured. You still had a duty to give her an honest answer.

As many patients are in shock when they have heard this news, it is possible that she may not have understood or remembered what you have said. Indeed many patients do not remember anything after being told that they have cancer. Therefore you should have ensured that the patient had understood everything you said.

'Mrs Patel, we have agreed to not go into any detail about your condition until your husband is present. However, I would like to make sure you have understood what I have said today and what is going to happen next. Could you perhaps summarise what we have said today? If it useful perhaps you could imagine that you are speaking to your husband. What would you tell him that we said?'

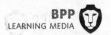

The patient should then hopefully re-iterate what you have told her correctly and you can end the consultation. Once again it is good practice to ask the patient if they have any questions before ending the consultation.

Notes

The important points in this consultation were to be sensitive and break the news to the patient in a way that was appropriate for her. In order to do this you needed to find out a little about what the patient expected, what she was concerned about and what she wanted to know. Therefore it was similar to the other consultations where we explored the patient's ideas, concerns and expectations. However, unlike the other consultations we did not need to spend a lot of time exploring the psychosocial aspect of her presenting complaint nor did we need to take a detailed history. We also did not need to go into great detail explaining the diagnosis, as we had done in our other consultations, simply because the patient did not wish to know all the details at this moment in time.

You did not need to use the SPIKES approach in your consultation. Some of you may have used your own approach or even used the other marking scheme we have used for our other consultations. The important thing was that you found out what the patient knew already, that you specifically elicited her concerns and her beliefs about what the results would show, and that you found how much information she wanted to know. Like the other consultations it was important to include them in making any management decisions and to take their feelings into consideration when making these decisions. Therefore, it was more about asking the patient what they wanted in advance, and then formulating a management plan with this is mind, as opposed to giving them several options to choose from as we have done before.

Unlike the other consultations, it is not as simple to decide if you have done well or not during the exercise. This is because these types of consultation are not about eliciting all the necessary information on the actor's brief. Consultations on breaking bad news focus more on your empathy and your ability to communicate clearly to the patient, tailoring your explanation to their individual needs. Therefore, it is very important in these types of consultations to get feedback from the actor on how you made them feel.

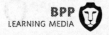

If the actor playing the patient did not feel comfortable or did not feel that you sympathised with how they felt, try to figure out why this was. Did you rush and give them too much information in one go? Did you not take the time to find out how much information they wanted to know and were ready to deal with? Perhaps you did not find out what they knew already and if they were expecting bad news? If this was the case replay the consultation specifically addressing these issues.

 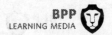

Mock Consultation 5

Doctor's brief

Mrs McCarthy is a 33-year-old lady who has come to you for her CT head result. She has been having persistent headaches for the past one month, which your colleague thought were tension headaches. As the headaches were not getting better, she was referred to see a Consultant Neurologist. The Consultant had seen her and although he could not find anything on examination, ordered a CT scan of her brain for completeness sake. The result of the scan is normal and she has been discharged from their care. You have never met her before.

Additional information

Mrs McCarthy's symptoms have not changed and she is still having headaches typical of a tension headache. There are no worrying features in the history or 'red-flag' symptoms. There is no need to examine the patient again or re-take the history.

You have 10 minutes to complete this task.

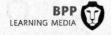

Use this space for your pre-consultation notes.

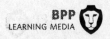

Mock Consultation 5

Patient's brief – *Do not read if you are playing the role of the doctor*

You are Mrs McCarthy, a 33-year-old woman, who has been having persistent headaches for the past one month. You were told by another GP in the practice that these were 'tension headaches'. However, after a month of no improvement you were concerned and demanded a referral to a Consultant Neurologist. He too could not find anything worrying on examination but ordered a scan of your brain for completeness sake. You have come today for the results of that scan.

Information unknown to the doctor

You are convinced you have a brain tumour. You were not satisfied by the diagnosis of 'tension headache' by the other GP and this is why you demanded a referral to a Consultant. You do not understand how a headache caused by stress or tension can be this bad, and you feel this is just an excuse used by the doctor because they do not know what is wrong with you. This is due to the fact that your sister died a year ago from a brain tumour which was misdiagnosed by the doctors. She too presented with persistent headaches and was told by her GP that everything was fine. When the tumour was diagnosed however, it was very large, and it was too late for her to have any treatment. As a result, you are mistrusting of doctors and are not reassured by the normal scan result, or that the Consultant could not find anything wrong on examination. At first you are quite upset and aggressive when the doctor tells you the scan is normal, and you make comments like, 'What you mean is *you* can't find anything wrong with me.' You are not willing to accept initially that the scan is normal and you do not have a tumour.

To make matters worse it is the month of the anniversary of your sister's death. You are very emotional right now and have not been coping well. You are not sleeping well, and although you do not feel depressed, you are feeling rather stressed at the moment. Work has also been quite testing and you are quite tired and run down. Your husband is also not being very supportive and thinks

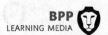

you are worrying over nothing. You are therefore very sensitive and become very angry if the doctor tries to imply that you are worrying for no reason.

However, if the doctor takes the time to explore your concerns, you are willing to accept the idea that perhaps the stress you are experiencing at the moment may be contributing to the headaches. If the doctor makes an effort to explain to you how stress can cause headaches, even persistent headaches, you accept the diagnosis completely. You decline any treatment for the headaches, feeling that now you are reassured, the headaches will stop. You also do not demand a second opinion.

However, if the doctor does not explore what has happened to make you feel so mistrusting and what is happening in your life right now, you will not accept anything they say about the scan being normal. You subsequently will not listen to anything they say and demand a second opinion.

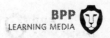

Mock Consultation 5

Information from brief

Things you may have picked up from the brief are:

Mrs McCarthy is a 33-year-old lady

This should prompt your thinking about what factors may be relevant in the consultation. As this implies she is married, it may be appropriate to discuss how things are going in her marriage or perhaps at work as she is of working age. The fact that she is 33 years of age shows she is relatively young which may be of importance later.

Who has come to you today for her CT head result

Here you should be considering what questions are relevant when explaining results to someone namely: establishing what they understand about why the test was being done, what they expect the results to be and what they understand by the test result you have given.

She has been having persistent headaches, for the past one month, which your colleague thought were tension headaches

This implies that she has been seen by another colleague. Therefore you should be wondering what your colleague explained to her and whether you need to ask her about this. It also states that she has been having the headaches for one month. This may be quite traumatic for anyone let alone a young 33-year-old woman who may be working and juggling a family. Therefore you should be thinking about this when exploring the psychosocial aspect of her presenting complaint. It also tells you that she has been diagnosed with 'tension headaches'. This raises two main issues: First, is she under stress at the moment hence why the diagnosis was made? Second, what does she understand by the term 'tension headache'?

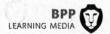

As the headaches were not getting better she was referred to see a Consultant Neurologist

This by itself does not mean much. However, it should raise the question as to why the referral was made. Was it because your colleague was unsure about the diagnosis? Or was it because the patient was not satisfied with the diagnosis and management plan given by the doctor? You may need to find this out later.

The Consultant had seen her and although he could not find anything on examination, ordered a CT scan of her brain for completeness sake

This is telling you that she has already been seen by a Consultant and little was found. Therefore you are unlikely to need to examine the patient again or take a further medical history. Also, you should be thinking about why the Consultant ordered a scan when he could find nothing on examination. Was it possibly because the patient needed reassurance? What was her understanding as to why he ordered the scan? Could it be possible that the fact a scan was ordered she feels there must be something wrong?

The result of the scan is normal and she has been discharged from their care

The scan is normal so you obviously need to explain this to the patient. However, the further management of this patient is in your hands as the Neurology team will not be seeing her again. Is the patient aware of this? How does she feel about this?

You have never met her before

You were initially told that she has seen your colleague. Now you are told that she has never met you before. Why is she coming to see you for the results when she has been under the care of one of your colleagues? Is it simply because you had the only available appointment? Could it be that perhaps she was not happy with the diagnosis and management suggested by your colleague?

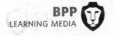

Mrs McCarthy's symptoms have not changed and she is still experiencing symptoms typical of a tension headache. There are no worrying features in the history or 'red-flag symptoms'. There is no need to examine the patient again or retake the history

This is telling you that there is no need to re-take a medical history and examine the patient. The history and examination has been done by your colleague as well as repeated by the Consultant Neurologist. It is also suggested that the diagnosis is a tension headache. You are specifically told that there are no new changes so you should not waste time on a history and examination.

In view of the fact that you are told you are not needed to make a new medical diagnosis there is likely to be an underlying issue that you need to explore.

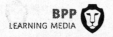

Mock Consultation 5

Suggested approach to the consultation by the doctor

1. **Creating a safe environment for the patient**

   This involves ensuring the furniture is adequately arranged and that there are no obstacles between you and the patient. You have never met this patient before and are suspecting that there is some underlying issue here that your colleague and the Consultant Neurologist have missed. Therefore, it will be particularly important to be in a position where you can see the patient as they are talking to pick up on any non-verbal clues they are giving you.

   As you have never met this patient before it will also be important to pay attention to your tone and body language. This is because the patient may not immediately feel comfortable with you, as they have never met you, and you will need to put them at ease. You will obviously also have needed to listen and show the patient that you were taking their concerns seriously.

   The actor's brief stated that at first the patient was quite aggressive and abrupt. It would have been important to not have reacted to this and to have stayed calm and let the patient voice their concerns.

2. **Introduction and opening statement**

   It is stated in the brief that you have never met the patient before. You should have made an effort to make her feel comfortable by inviting her in, calling her by her name, and introducing yourself.

   Although you are told the reason for her presentation in the brief you should have asked her an open question as your opening statement. This would allow you to pick up on any clues she was giving you and enable you to gain more information from the patient than a simple 'yes' or 'no' answer would.

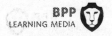

> *'Mrs McCarthy, please come in and have a seat. I don't believe we have met before? I am Dr Clark. How can I help today?'*

Some of you may have made reference to the fact that she had seen your colleague before in the opening statement, e.g.

> *'Mrs McCarthy. I don't believe we have met before? I am Dr Clark, I believe you saw one of my colleagues last time?'*

This is perfectly acceptable as long as it is followed by an open question such as 'How can I help today?', or something similar. This is simple because asking her if she saw one of your colleagues can only be answered by a 'yes' or 'no' and may not elicit any more information.

The patient may then reply with:

> *'Yes I saw your colleague about a month ago as I was having these headaches. I went for a scan and I have come for the results.'*

You may then need to go on from your opening statement and ask the patient what your colleague had discussed with them and what they were expecting the scan to show. This will allow you to get a better perspective of what the patient understands about their symptoms so far and what they are expecting. Therefore if the patient does not mention that she has seen your colleague and the Consultant previously, it would be important to specifically mention this and ask her what she has been told.

3. **Encourage the patient's contribution at appropriate points in the consultation**
   This describes active listening and may have included nodding as she was talking or perhaps acknowledging what she was saying with a 'hmm'. It may have also involved encouraging her to go on if you felt she was hesitating or was unsure of whether to continue. In these circumstances you may have said to the patient:

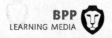

> • *'Please continue Mrs McCarthy.'*
> • *'Really? Tell me more?'*

You may have also tried to encourage her to talk a little more after she simply said that she had come for her scan results. You may have asked her to tell you a little more about what has been happening over the last month. Or you may have asked her to tell you what happened when she saw your colleague in more detail.

You may have also used the skill of reflecting back, where you repeat what the patient said with a pause, in the hope that they will continue explaining, for example:

> • *'You said you are worried . . .'*
> • *'You said you were not convinced by the results . . .'*

Hopefully the patient will then continue the sentence and explain what she meant by those comments and you will have encouraged her to reveal her agenda.

4. **Respond to cues that lead to a deeper understanding of the problem**
   This may have involved picking up on any verbal or non-verbal clues the patient was giving you. In the actor's brief they were specifically told to come across quite aggressive when you reveal that the scan results are normal. This is a major clue and should alert you to the fact that there is a reason behind her not being satisfied with the result. The patient was also told to make a comment along the lines of:

> *'Actually what you mean doctor is **you** can't find anything wrong with me. Just because the scan is normal, it does not necessarily mean that there is not something wrong with me, does it?'*

Obviously this is another major clue and you should have picked up and commented on this to the patient. Therefore you may have made comments like:

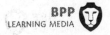

> - *'You don't seem to be reassured by the normal scan result. Would I be correct in saying so?'*
> - *'When you said that a normal scan did not mean that there was not something wrong with you, what did you mean by that?'*

Although the patient may be coming across quite upset and abrupt at this point it is important to not let this distract you or to become annoyed with the patient. Try to stay calm and simply empathise with the patient, reflecting back what they are saying or how they are coming across, to gain a deeper understanding. You will be surprised by how simply doing this can often calm patients down and encourage them to reveal to you what they are really worried about.

Therefore in this brief the patient may say something like:

> - *'No I am not reassured by the result. I know that sometimes doctors get it wrong. I know that first hand.'*
> - *'Well doctor sometimes you are told that everything is okay but it really isn't. So to me a normal scan does not mean much. They could have got it wrong.'*

Obviously these comments need to be explored in more detail and you would need to enquire why the patient feels that way. This would be exploring the patient's ideas, concerns and expectations which we will discuss shortly.

5. **Elicit appropriate details to place the complaints in a social and psychosocial context**
When reading the brief we already thought about the impact a chronic headache would have on a patient. To be able to get a deeper insight into how it is affecting this particular patient, we need to ask the relevant questions. As the brief states she is 33 years old, and implies she is married, you should have asked her how this is affecting her home and work life. Therefore you may have asked her:

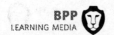

> • *'How is this headache affecting you? Does it stop you from doing anything you want to do?'*
> • *'Have you been able to cope at work with this headache?'*
> • *'Who is with you at home? How does your husband feel about this?'*

The patient may then have revealed that she is under stress at work and home and not sleeping well.

> *'Well to be honest doctor I am extremely stressed out at the moment. Work is difficult enough without having a constant headache. My husband is at home with me but he hasn't been too helpful at the moment . . .'*

This is again an obviously clue which you would have needed to pick up on at some point:

> *'Mrs McCarthy, you said your husband was not very helpful at the moment. What did you mean by that?'*

This may have prompted her to tell you the information in the brief: that her husband thinks she is worrying over nothing and that she is not happy about this.

> *'Well, he thinks I am just stressed and there is nothing wrong with me. Your colleague thought that as well. He told me I have a tension headache.'*

Again, the patient is giving you a clue here especially as she is using medical terminology. You should have explored what she understood by that term and went on to explore her health understanding.

6. **Explore the patient's health understanding**
   This involves exploring the patient's health beliefs, the things that are concerning them as well as what they expected from the consultation today. This often ties in closely with picking up on clues that the patient has given you, as these are usually clues as to what the patient believes or is worried about.

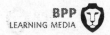

Therefore, by picking up on certain clues already you may have gathered that patient is still anxious and is not reassured by the normal scan result. If you had done this you could have reflected this back to the patient, commenting that you had noticed she seems worried or commenting on what she had said, and asking her why she feels this way. If you had not picked up on her anxiety already, by asking the patient what it was she was worried about and what she thought was wrong with her, you should have definitely realised that there was an issue. Therefore, you should have asked the patient about their health beliefs.

> • 'Mrs McCarthy. Patients often have an idea as to what could be causing their symptoms. What do you think is causing these headaches?'
> • 'What is your main fear about these headaches? Is there any particular condition you are worrying that they represent?'
> • 'What were you hoping would happen today?'
> • 'What were you expecting the scan to show today?'
> • 'What do you understand by "tension headache"?'

The patient should have then hopefully told you that she was worried she had a brain tumour. She may have told you why she felt this way straight away or you may have had to delve a little deeper.

> 'Well, doctor, I don't believe these are "tension headaches" as your colleague has told me. I have a headache and I have been stressed before and never had a headache. So why is it happening now? I know people say stress can cause a lot of things but I don't believe it would cause such a bad headache. I am worried really that I have a brain tumour. I know my scan is normal but I want a second opinion.'

This has given you quite a large amount of information and you are now aware of what the patient is worried about. However, it is slightly unusual for a young 33-year-old patient to be worried about a brain tumour, and therefore it is important to enquire why this is. Again this is picking up on a clue, and

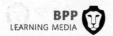

it is useful to use the process of clarifying and reflecting back this clue to the patient to understand what is going on.

> *'You said you are worried about a brain tumour? I can understand that must be quite worrying for you. Is there any particular reason why you feel that it is a tumour?'*

The patient may then have told you about her sister being diagnosed with a brain tumour after being told everything was okay:

> *'Well my sister had headaches for absolutely ages. She went to the doctors so many times and they kept telling her everything was okay. Next thing I knew she is being told it's a tumour, but it was too large to remove as it was found too late. She died shortly after.'*

Giving you this information is likely to be very upsetting for the patient and you should have responded with an empathic comment when you were told this:

> - *'That must have come as a big shock to you. When did all this happen?'*
> - *'I'm so sorry to hear that. This must be very difficult for you to discuss.'*

The patient may then have told you that this happened this time last year and give you more details into the circumstances with her sister. This has now given you a major clue as to what may be causing her reluctance to accept the results, and what may be making her even more anxious. It is therefore useful to have suggested this to the patient:

> *'Mrs McCarthy, I appreciate it must be very upsetting for you to have lost your sister so suddenly like that and frightening for you now that you are experiencing similar symptoms around the same time of year. Do you think that the fact that your sister was told there was nothing wrong with her is making you more suspicious that there is something going on with you that we have missed?'*

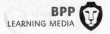

The patient may have perhaps agreed with you or may have even denied it depending on the actor. The important thing is that you suggested that what happened with her sister may be worsening how she feels and did not imply that she is imagining it or making it up. This is only likely to have upset the patient even more. The patient may have responded with something like this:

> 'Well I never really thought of it that way. I guess I am more sceptical about doctors since my sister's diagnosis, but I am still getting headaches and I am worried about them. My husband thinks that I am worrying over nothing but I know how I feel.'

7. **Obtain sufficient information to include or exclude likely relevant significant conditions**
    You are already told that you do need to take a medical history in this case. Some of you may have not trusted the information in the brief and may have asked her if anything had changed since she was last seen. This is perfectly appropriate as long as you simply asked this and did not try and take the history again. Some of you may also have asked her a few more questions to try and gain more insight into her mental state at this time, considering what she has told you about her sister. Do not worry if you did not ask them, they were not necessary for this consultation.

    > - 'Have you been sleeping?'
    > - 'Have you been eating?'
    > - 'Have you been feeling tearful?'
    > - 'Have you had any thoughts of harming yourself?'

8. **Choose an appropriate physical or mental examination**
    You are specifically told that you do not need to examine the patient in this consultation so this is irrelevant.

9. **Make a clinically appropriate working diagnosis/explain the diagnosis to the patient in appropriate language taking into account the patient's elicited beliefs**
    This should have involved explaining the scan results to the patient fully and what you thought was causing her headaches.

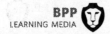

The headache is real to the patient, and you should have been careful to not come across as patronising.

> • *'Mrs McCarthy, you told me earlier that you are worried you have a brain tumour. Although, I appreciate that sometimes mistakes are made I think it is very unlikely that we have missed a tumour. For one, you have not had any worrying symptoms that may suggest a tumour and when we examined you we did not notice any nerve damage that would be caused by a tumour. However, as you stated doctors can sometimes makes mistakes. However, the fact that you have had a normal scan result excludes a brain tumour completely. This is because a scan is very sensitive to this sort of problem and we would have definitely seen the tumour on the scan.'*
> • *'I do appreciate however, that this is a very bad time of year for you right now, with the anniversary of your sister's death and your work stresses. You mentioned earlier that the previous doctor had told you that you had a "tension headache" I think that this is likely the cause. Do you understand what we mean by a "tension headache"?'*
> • *'You also mentioned that you didn't understand how stress can cause such a bad headache. Well when we are stressed the muscles in our head and neck can become very tight and this causes pain. This can be very frightening which often causes us to worry more. This in turn causes the muscles to become even tenser and this can often become a vicious circle making the headache prolonged. Does this make sense?'*

This is making an effort to specifically reassure the patient that it is not a tumour, but it also going into more depth about what a tension headache is to allow the patient to understand that this diagnosis could explain her symptoms.

10. **Make an appropriate management plan/involve the patient in significant management decisions**
Your plan may vary and once again please remember that you will not score any marks for your management plan. What you will be marked on however is including the patient in any management decisions you have made. Some of you may have offered her pain relief, some may have offered counselling. Some may have offered her specific medication for chronic

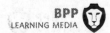

tension headaches such as amitryptiline. Others may have offered a 'watch and wait' policy. The important thing is to give her the choice in what to do.

> *'They are several ways we can treat tension headaches. The options are that you could try a painkiller to see if this helps with the pain. You could also try non-medical therapies such as massage and relaxation techniques to see if this helps relax the muscles in the head and relieve the pain. We could also just wait and see if the headache goes away by itself. If this doesn't help I can always refer you for a second opinion. I could also refer you immediately for a second opinion as you had requested earlier. However, I am confident that if we try some simple pain relief and relaxation techniques the headaches will improve. What would you like to do?'*

The patient was specifically told to accept your management plan if you had explained everything properly and adequately reassured her. So hopefully she should have agreed to try something for the pain and not demanded a referral. Had she still demanded a referral for a second opinion, you obviously did not listen to the patient or address her issues.

11. **When prescribing take steps to enhance concordance by exploring and responding to the patient's understanding of the treatment**
Unless you are prescribing this point is not relevant. If you have prescribed medication, it may be useful to explain the side effects and how the patient takes them. In a case like this where there are so many issues you will probably only have time to briefly mention it:

> *'We have decided to try some ibuprofen. This is a painkiller which also helps reduce any inflammation in the muscles around the head. You should take it regularly; as if you only take it occasionally it may not work as well. Therefore I would like you to take it three times a day preferably with something to eat. Unfortunately it can cause indigestion problems, so if you do experience any discomfort in your tummy or indigestion please stop the tablets and let me know.'*

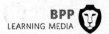

Once again, do not worry too much about this point; it is unlikely to gain you many extra marks. It may be more appropriate in other cases however which focus much more on prescribing.

12. **Specify the conditions and interval for follow up and review (safety net)**

Although the scan has come back normal, and you are sure this is a tension headache, you could be wrong. Also as the patient is concerned it may also reassure her to offer her some follow up or a back-up plan should things worsen.

> *'Mrs McCarthy, I would like to see you in two weeks to see how you are progressing and if the headaches have improved. Is that okay with you? In the meantime if the headaches should worsen or you experience any pain looking at lights or a stiff neck, I would like you to see a doctor immediately.'*

It is important to not be reluctant to safety-net with patients who were initially anxious. If you have explained things properly and sufficiently reassured them you will not panic them by safety-netting. Therefore, you must ensure you safety-net in each case.

13. **Confirm the patient's understanding**

Here you needed to have ensured that the patient understood everything you said. Therefore you may have ask her to summarise what you have said to ensure she understood.

> *'Just so I can make sure we have both understood each other today could you please summarise what we have said today and what we are going to do?'*

Again, the patient should have clearly summarised what has been said in the consultation if you have been clear in your communication.

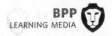

> 'The results of my scan have come back normal and it is therefore
> very unlikely that I have a tumour. You think I have a tension
> headache which is caused by the muscles of the head becoming
> tense. I have probably been worrying because of what happened
> to my sister and I have been stressed at work. I am going to try
> taking regular ibuprofen for two weeks and then come back to
> see you. If I get worse in the meantime however I should come
> back sooner.'

You should have then ended the consultation by asking the
patient if they had any more questions and thanking them.

Notes

The actor is specifically told in their brief that if you have explored
their sister's death and have sympathised with how they are feeling,
they will agree with your diagnosis. Therefore, if the actor did not
agree with your diagnosis, it is likely because you did not explore
the patient's feelings enough or did not listen to the patient. It
may have also been because you did not handle their aggression
well and perhaps antagonised the patient by becoming aggravated
yourself. Ask the observer and the patient what went wrong and
then replay the consultation using some of the approaches we
have discussed.

They were also told that they will only accept the diagnosis of a
tension headache if you explain to them what it is and how it is
caused. This shows the importance of communication and it may
be that your colleague before did not explain how such a simple
diagnosis could explain her symptoms. Therefore, if the patient
queried your diagnosis or still demanded a second opinion ask
the actor why this was. Was it because you were not sympathetic
enough? Or was it because you did not explain to them what a
tension headache was and how the stress she was experiencing
could have prolonged the headache and made it worse? Once again
replay the consultation at this point to see if explaining things in
more detail could change the outcome of the consultation.

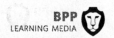

Mock Consultation 6

Doctor's brief

Miss Lemming, a 30-year-old lady, has come to see you today to discuss her periods. She has been having irregular periods for just over two months now, only having one period in the last two months. She previously had normal periods. She therefore saw your colleague about three weeks ago who requested a pelvic ultrasound scan and some baseline blood tests. All the blood tests including her prolactin levels, thyroid function and gonadotrophin levels have come back as normal. The pelvic ultrasound scan was also normal. Miss Lemming saw your colleague about two weeks ago who reassured her about the results. She has still however not had a period.

Additional information

Miss Lemming is not on any form of contraception and has already had a pregnancy test which was negative. She is currently not sexually active. Previously she has always had normal periods and has no family history of note. Her smears are up to date and she has also had vaginal swabs to exclude any infection. The history has not changed and there is no need to examine the patient.

You have 10 minutes to complete this task.

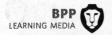

Use this space for your pre-consultation notes.

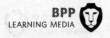

Mock Consultation 6

Patient's brief – *Do not read if you are playing the role of the doctor*

> Your name is Miss Lemming and you are a 30-year-old lady who has been having irregular periods for two months now. You have only had one period in the last two months. Previously your periods were always regular and everything was fine. You came to see another GP who requested some blood tests and a scan of your pelvis. These have all come back as normal and you were reassured that there was no medical cause for your irregular periods.

Information unknown to the doctor

You are a naturally very anxious patient and give the GP clues from the start that you are worried. You have been under a lot of stress recently as you broke up with your boyfriend about five months ago. You were together for ten years and you took the break up very badly. You do not reveal this information unless the doctor specifically asks you about your personal life and how things have been in the past few months.

You have subsequently not been eating or sleeping well, and have lost about half a stone in the past five months. You have good social support and get on well with your family and friends who are being supportive. Although you feel quite down at times, you are not suicidal and are managing to still go to work daily. You enjoy your job and feels it takes your mind off your personal problems.

Your main concern is that you are worried you will never have children. You were convinced that you and your ex-partner would get married and start a family. Now that you are single again at 30, you are wondering if this will ever happen. You secretly believe that your irregular periods are a sign of an early menopause and are worried that it may mean that you are going to become infertile. Unless the doctor specifically reassures you that this is not the case, you remain anxious and unsatisfied by their advice.

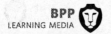

If the doctor is sympathetic to how you feel and reassures you that you are not going through an early menopause, you are open to the suggestion that it may be the stress and weight loss that has upset your periods. However, if the doctor has not listened to you or taken steps to reassure you, you refuse to listen to anything they say and leave the room.

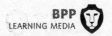

Mock Consultation 6

Information from the brief

Things you may have picked up from the brief are:

Miss Lemming, a 30-year-old lady, has come to see you today to discuss her periods

The patient is relatively young and her name implies that she is not married. In view of her presenting complaint of irregular periods this may be relevant. As she is young it will make menopause very unlikely, however it is also not usual to suddenly start having irregular periods as 30. Therefore, as you are told the medical tests are all normal you should have started thinking about what else could be causing this. You should also have started thinking about what psychosocial questions may be relevant to a patient of this age.

She has been having irregular periods for just over two months now, only having one period in the last two months. She previously had normal periods

Although this may be worrying for the patient it is not from a medical perspective a long time to go without a period. Is the patient aware that some women can miss two periods without there being a serious medical cause? However, you should have also started thinking about why the patient may feel anxious that this has happened, especially when she had regular periods previously. You should also have started thinking about what things could have caused her periods to become suddenly irregular.

She therefore saw your colleague about three weeks ago who requested a pelvic ultrasound scan and some baseline blood tests. All the blood tests including her prolactin levels, thyroid function and gonadotrophin levels have all come back as normal. The pelvic ultrasound was also normal

This should have prompted you thinking about what else could have caused her irregular periods as all the medical tests are negative. You should have also been thinking about whether the patient understood what tests had been done and what conditions had

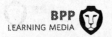

been excluded. As you are well aware that stress and psychological problems can affect the menstrual cycle you should have also been prepared to ask her questions on this.

She has seen your colleague two weeks ago who reassured her about the results

This should have encouraged you to consider why the patient has come to see you when she has already been reassured by your colleague. You may have suspicions about either a hidden agenda or perhaps a lack of sympathy or explanation on your colleague's part. There has to be a reason as to why she has come back.

She has still not had a period

This should have raised the question as to whether this was the reason that she was coming back to see you. Is she still not reassured and therefore still worried as she has not had a period since she was seen two weeks ago? Or perhaps she was told to come back if she did not have a period in the next two weeks? What are her expectations as to when her periods should return?

Additional information

This information is simply telling you that every possible medical cause for her irregular periods have been excluded so there is no need to take a medical history or examine the patient.

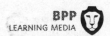

Mock Consultation 6

Suggested approach to the consultation by the doctor

1. **Creating a safe environment for the patient**

- *Was the furniture appropriately placed so that there were no obstacles between you and the patient?*
- *The patient was meant to have come across as quite anxious when she walked in. Were you at an appropriate distance and angle to be able to see the patient's non-verbal expressions?*
- *How were you seated? Was your body language appropriate? How did your body language make the patient feel? Did they feel comfortable?*
- *As the patient was anxious, did you keep a soft sympathetic tone when talking to the patient? Did you empathise with the patient at the appropriate points?*

2. **Introduction and opening statement**

- *Did you greet the patient using the name that was given in the brief?*
- *Did you introduce who you were?*
- *Did you comment on the fact that she had seen your colleague before?*
- *Did you use an open question when asking the patient what brought her to see you today?*
- *After the patient told you why she had come today, did you take steps to ask her what she had discussed with your colleague previously? Did you ask her to explain what she understood about what tests were done and why?*

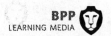

3. **Encourage the patient's contribution at appropriate points in the consultation**

> • *Did you take active steps to show the patient you were listening, e.g. nodding your head, maintaining eye contact?*
> • *Did you encourage the patient to continue if she paused or had difficulty revealing the information to you?*
>
> • *Did you show empathy if the patient found it difficult talking about certain things or was anxious to tell you how she felt?*

e.g. *'I understand this must be difficult for you.'*

> *If the patient was initially reluctant to tell you what was worrying her, did you leave it at that or did you try to pursue the matter? If you pursued this further, did you do this appropriately and sensitively? Or did you directly keep asking her questions that you could see she was uncomfortable answering?*

4. **Respond to cues that lead to a deeper understanding of the problem**

> *Did you pick up that the patient was very anxious and reflect this back to the patient?*

e.g. *'You seem very anxious today.'*

> *Did you watch the patient carefully to look for non-verbal clues? Did you comment to the patient on what you had noticed?*

e.g. *'You seem to be a little upset.'*

> • *Did you listen to the patient without interrupting to be able to pick up on any hints she was giving you?*
> • *Did you pick up on these clues and either reflect them back to the patient or ask her to clarify them, in order to gain a deeper insight into how she felt?*

e.g. *'You said earlier that you know you will never have any children. What did you mean by that?'*

5. Elicit appropriate details to place the complaints in a social and psychosocial context

- *The patient was specifically having a problem dealing with the break-up of a relationship. Did you elicit that information? If not, why not? Did you ask her if she was in a relationship at the moment or who was at home with her? You are told in the brief that she is not sexually active. Is this because she is not in a relationship? Or could it be due to problems in a current relationship?*
- *If she revealed that she was not in a relationship, but gave you a clue to the fact that she was recently in one, did you explore this further? Did you explore how the break-up had affected her?*
- *Did you specifically ask the patient how the worry over her periods was affecting her? As she was obviously very anxious did you ask if this anxiety was stopping her from eating, sleeping or affecting her work life?*

6. Explore the patient's health understanding

- *Considering the patient was very anxious did you ask her what she was worried these irregular periods represented or what could be causing them?*
- *Did you ask the patient what she expected the test results to show?*
- *Did you ask the patient what she understood by your colleague telling her the tests results were normal? Did she understand what diagnoses had been excluded?*
- *Did you pick up on the fact that the patient was worried she was going through an early menopause. If not, why was that? Did you ask the correct questions to elicit her ideas and concerns? Were you sympathetic when you asked these questions?*
- *Did you ask her what she expected to happen today? Did she want a referral to a specialist or was she looking for a second opinion and reassurance from yourself?*

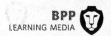

7. **Obtain sufficient information to include or exclude likely relevant significant conditions**

> - *You were told in the brief that the medical history had not changed and therefore you did not need to take a gynaecological history. Did you pay attention to the brief or did you start asking numerous questions about her periods?*
> - *If you wanted to clarify the information in the brief, did you do this by simply asking if anything had changed since she was last seen or did you take a full gynaecological history?*
> - *In view of the patient being very anxious and revealing to you she is stressed, did you ask a few questions to exclude depression? Did you make sure she was not suicidal?*
> - *If she told you she wasn't eating well. Did you ask her if she had lost weight? Did you ask her how much weight she had lost being aware that dramatic weight loss can affect the menstrual cycle?*

8. **Choose an appropriate physical or mental examination**

> *Did you waste time examining the patient or did you pay attention to the brief which stated that an examination of the patient was not necessary?*

9. **Make a clinically appropriate working diagnosis / explain the diagnosis to the patient in appropriate language taking into account the patient's elicited beliefs**

> - *Did you explain to the patient what you thought was causing her irregular periods in simple language?*
> - *Did you suggest sensitively to the patient that perhaps her break up from her partner and the stress she has been under has triggered off her irregular periods?*
> - *Did you explain to her how stress and weight loss can affect the menstrual cycle?*
> - *Did you take active steps to specifically reassure her that this was not an early menopause and that the blood tests had completely ruled that out? Did you actively reassure*

> *her that this did not mean that she was infertile and could never have children?*
> - *Did you reassure the patient that her periods should come back to normal once she regains some weight and starts to become less stressed?*

10. Make an appropriate management plan / involve the patient in significant management decisions

> - *Once again the exact nature of your management plan was not important. What was important is that you included the patient in the decision making process. Therefore did you ask the patient what she thought would be best for her?*
> - *Did you involve the patient in whatever management decision you made?*
> - *What did your management plan involve? Did it involve simply watching and waiting? Or did you offer her any help and support to help her through this stressful time? If you did not offer her any support why was this? Was it because you focussed too much on the medical aspect of her presenting complaint?*
> - *Did the patient seem happy with what you had suggested? If not was this because you did not take her beliefs into account when making these management decisions? Or was it because she did not feel reassured by your diagnosis and explanation.*

11. When prescribing take steps to enhance concordance by exploring and responding to the patient's understanding of the treatment

> - *As you are unlikely to have prescribed anything in this scenario this point is not relevant.*
> - *However, had you prescribed any medication such as sleeping tablets, did you take steps to explain to the patient how they worked and addressed any concerns they had about the medication?*

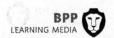

12. **Specify the conditions and interval for follow up and review (safety net)**

> - *Did you offer the patient another appointment should her periods have not have returned by a certain point?*
>
> - *Did you suggest to the patient that perhaps you might refer her to a gynaecologist should her periods not have returned in a few months?*
> - *Did you inform the patient that should her mood deteriorate and she finds herself not coping that she should come back to see you as soon as possible?*

13. **Confirm the patient's understanding**

> - *Did you actively take steps to ensure the patient had understood what you had said?*
> - *Did you ask her to summarise what you had said? Did the patient summarise the information correctly?*

Notes

The patient was told to leave the room if you had not taken steps to reassure her that she was not going through an early menopause. Therefore, if the consultation went wrong and the patient became upset or walked out, it is likely to be because you did not address the patient's concerns. This may be because you forgot to ask her about what she was worried about or perhaps because you were not paying enough attention to pick up on the clues she was giving you. If this happened to you, replay the consultation spending more time exploring the patient's ideas, concerns and expectations, and see if this changes the outcome of the consultation.

Once again, it was fundamental to have addressed the psychosocial aspect of her presenting complaint in order to understand why she was worried and what had triggered this all off. Therefore you should have asked her about whether she was in a relationship or explored her social background in order to give her the opportunity to tell you that she had recently broken up with someone. Although this may seem artificial it is good practice to ask about relationships

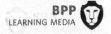

in all of your consultations. Therefore, even if you picked up that she was worried about an early menopause, if you did not find out about her break up, you would not have been able to truly empathise with the patient as to why she was so worried. Once again, if this was the case replay the consultation, this time concentrating more on the social aspect of the patient's life and asking her specific questions about how things are going.

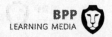

Mock Consultation 7

Doctor's brief

Mr Buchanan is a 37-year-old gentleman who has come to see you for his endoscopy results. He is a relatively new patient, having only been with your surgery for the past three months. He had been referred for the endoscopy as he was complaining of persistent epigastric pain, despite being on omeprazole. He has no red flags such as weight loss, appetite loss, melaena or haematemesis. The results of the endoscopy including the CLO test are all normal.

Additional information

Prior to the endoscopy Mr Buchanan also had an ultrasound of his abdomen which was normal. He also had bloods including a full blood count, liver function test and amylase which were also normal. He was already informed about these results and there is no need to inform him about these again. The history has not changed and he still has no red flag symptoms. There is no need to examine the patient.

You have 10 minutes to complete this task.

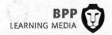

Use this space for your pre-consultation notes.

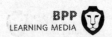

Mock Consultation 7

Patient's brief – *Do not read if you are playing the role of the doctor*

> You are Mr Buchanan, a 37-year-old gentleman, who has come for your endoscopy results. The test was done as you were getting persistent pains in your stomach. You had been put on omeprazole to see if this helped your symptoms but it only helped slightly. You also had an ultrasound scan of your abdomen which was also normal.

Information unknown to the doctor

You work in the city as an investment banker and have an extremely stressful job. You come across as having a 'type A' personality and can be quite intimidating. You are very highly driven but do put yourself under a lot of pressure. When you are told the results are normal you become quite vocal, asking the doctor in a very stern manner if he is sure that there is nothing wrong. You are convinced that you have a stomach ulcer, as you were diagnosed with this previously about eight years ago, and feel your symptoms are the same. Therefore you will not be easily convinced that the results are normal and need specific reassurance that you do not have a stomach ulcer.

You are aware that excess alcohol can cause an irritation of the stomach and are drinking in excess of your recommended allowance of 21 units a week. This is mainly due to hosting working lunches with clients, but also due to being lonely at home in the evenings, where you can have half a bottle of wine a night. You have broken-up from your wife a year ago and have been feeling very down in the evenings. You are secretly concerned about your drinking, which is the real reason you had come to the doctor in the first place, but were too embarrassed to admit it. You think that your drinking, combined with the stress you are under, is the real reason for the pains you are having.

You are very reluctant to reveal the information about your drinking to the doctor, and will only do so if he asks you about your work and home life in detail. You initially reveal very little, just giving

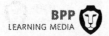

the doctor a hint that your job involves hosting daily lunches with clients where you have the 'odd occasional drink'. You come across as quite embarrassed to talk about this and try to play down how much you drink at work saying 'it's not much'. You only reveal how much you truly drink if the doctor explores this further, and specifically asks how much you drink a day or week.

If the doctor tries to address your drinking without exploring the reasons behind it and being sympathetic to how you are feeling, you react very badly. You accuse the doctor of calling you an alcoholic and get very annoyed. However, if the doctor elicits the information regarding your break-up from your wife, and sympathises with how difficult it must have been for you, you are then open to any suggestions he gives you.

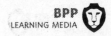

Mock Consultation 7

Information from brief

Things you may have picked up from the brief are:

Mr Buchanan is a 37-year-old gentleman who has come to see you for his endoscopy results

As you are given his age in the brief this is likely to be relevant at some point. Therefore you should have started thinking about what psychosocial questions may be relevant to a 37 year old. As he is of working age you should therefore have considered asking him about his occupation. As he is coming to see you for his endoscopy results you should have been wondering about what he understood about why the test was done and what he expected it to show.

He is a new patient

This may be relevant in that you may not have all the patient's previous records to hand. Therefore it may be important to ask him about if he has had any similar problems in the past and his past medical history.

He had been referred for the endoscopy as he was complaining of persistent epigastric pain despite being on omeprazole

This seems a sensible reason to refer someone for an endoscopy. However, did the patient understand why he was being referred? What did he expect the results to find?

He had no red flags such as weight loss, appetite loss, melaena or haematemesis

This makes it unlikely that anything sinister is going on. Also the fact that you are being told this in the brief means you are unlikely to have to about these again in your consultation.

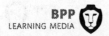

The results of the endoscopy including the CLO test are all normal

You are told that the results are normal. Is the patient still having pains? If so what could be causing this in view of the normal results?

Additional information

The additional information is confirming once again that you have excluded a medical cause for this pain. It is also telling you that the history has not changed and therefore there is no need to take a full medical history again. It also clearly tells you that there is no need to examine the patient.

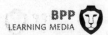

Mock Consultation 7

Suggested approach to the consultation by the doctor

1. Creating a safe environment for the patient

- *Was the furniture appropriately placed so there were no obstacles between you and the patient?*
- *The patient was meant to have come across as quite intimidating. Did you leave an appropriate distance between you and the patient, or were you seated too close? Did the patient then have to move his chair back or did you have to move back from the patient because it felt uncomfortable? Were you close enough however to see the patient's non-verbal expressions?*
- *How did you react when this patient became intimidating? Did you raise your voice to overpower the patient? Or did you remain calm?*
- *What was your body language like? Did you become defensive when the patient was aggressive? Or did you pay particular attention to not be threatening yourself to the patient? How did the patient feel by your mannerisms? Did you manage to calm the patient down?*
- *Did you empathise with the patient? If he told you about the problems he was having did you show sympathy encouraging him to open up more?*

2. Introduction and opening statement

- *Did you greet the patient using the name that was given in the brief?*
- *Did you introduce who you were?*
- *Did you use an open question when asking the patient what had brought him to see you today?*
- *After the patient has told you why he had come today did you take steps to ask him what he understood as to why the endoscopy was requested?*

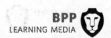

3. **Encourage the patient's contribution at appropriate points in the consultation**

> - *Did you take active steps to show the patient you were listening, e.g. nodding your head, maintaining eye contact?*
> - *Did you encourage the patient to continue if he paused or had difficulty revealing the information to you?*
> - *Did you pick on the clue that the patient was embarrassed to talk about his drinking? Did you encourage him to tell you more about this in a sensitive manner?*

4. **Respond to cues that lead to a deeper understanding of the problem**

> - *Did you pick up on the clue that the patient gave you about his drinking when he told you that he often drinks at work? Did you explore this further by asking how much he drinks? Did you ask him by what he meant by 'not a lot' in response to how much he drinks?*
> - *Did you pick up on the fact that he tried to play this fact down and seemed a bit embarrassed to discuss it?*

e.g. *'You seem a bit reluctant to talk to me about how much you drink, would I be correct in saying so?'*

> - *Did you pick up on the fact that the patient had a type 'A' personality and was prone to a lot of stress? Based on this did you ask him if he was under a lot of stress at the moment?*
> - *Did you listen to the patient without interrupting to be able to pick up on any hints he was giving you?*
> - *Did you pick up on these clues and either reflect them back to the patient or ask him to clarify them, in order to gain a deeper insight into how he felt?*

e.g. *'You mentioned that you think you may have a stomach ulcer, can you tell me what you mean by that?'*

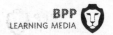

5. **Elicit appropriate details to place the complaints in a social and psychosocial context**
This was the key to understanding the case.

> - *Did you ask the patient about his occupation?*
> - *Did you ask the patient if this pain affected his work? If so he may have given you a clue that he was a workaholic who let little affect his work.*
> - *Did you ask him what his job entails? Did he tell you that it is stressful and often involves working lunches with clients?*
> - *Did you ask him who was with him at home or if he was married? If so he may have revealed to you that he had broken-up with his wife.*
> - *If he revealed his break-up to you did you explore how he was coping with the situation? If you had done so he may have revealed to you that he drinks to cope with the loneliness.*
> - *Did you ask him who he turns to for support? Did he tell you that he is quite alone and turns to alcohol to help ease his worries?*

6. **Explore the patient's health understanding**

> - *Did you ask the patient specifically what he expected the results to show?*
> - *If he mentioned that he suspected the endoscopy would show an ulcer, did you ask him why that was? Did he then reveal to you that this was because he had an ulcer before and is having similar pains?*
> - *Did you ask him if he had any ideas what else could be causing his pain? If so he may have revealed that he thought the alcohol and stress may have been causing the pain.*
> - *Did you ask him what he was concerned this pain may represent? Did he tell you that he was concerned it may be a sign he is drinking too much? If not why didn't he tell you? Had you listened to the patient and been sympathetic throughout?*

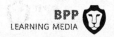

7. **Obtain sufficient information to include or exclude likely relevant significant conditions**

- *You were told in the brief that the medical history had not changed and therefore you did not need to retake the history. Did you pay attention to the brief or did you start asking numerous questions about his pain?*
- *Did you enquire as to whether he was still having these epigastric pains?*
- *Did you ask him if anything had changed since he was last seen? This would have confirmed that the information in the brief was correct.*
- *Did you explore his alcohol intake further? For example, did you ask him exactly how much he drank so that you could quantify how bad the problem was?*
- *Did you perhaps use a screening tool such as the CAGE questionnaire to screen for alcoholism i.e.*
  - *Do you ever feel you should cut down on your drinking?*
  - *Do you ever become angry/annoyed when others mention your drinking?*
  - *Do you ever feel guilty about your drinking?*
  - *Do you ever have drink first thing in the morning to steady your nerves or help your hangover (Eye-opener)?*

8. **Choose an appropriate physical or mental examination**

If the patient admitted that he was still having these pains in his epigastrium did you offer to examine the patient's abdomen later? If you did not offer to examine him, do not worry as the brief did state there was no need to examine the patient. However, it would have been good practice to have offered to re-examine him.

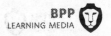

9. **Make a clinically appropriate working diagnosis / explain the diagnosis to the patient in appropriate language taking into account the patient's elicited beliefs**

> - *Did you explain to the patient that the results of the endoscopy were normal and you had definitely excluded an ulcer?*
> - *Did you explain to the patient that you agreed that perhaps the excess drinking and the stress he was under could be causing his pains?*
> - *Did you explain how stress and alcohol can cause stomach pains? If you did this, was it in simple language that the patient could understand?*
> - *Did you sympathise with how difficult it must be coping with the break-up from his wife and a stressful job when you gave your explanation?*
> - *Did you clearly inform the patient that he was drinking above his recommended allowance and that this needed to be addressed?*

10. **Make an appropriate management plan / involve the patient in significant management decisions**

> - *Did you involve the patient in whatever management decision you made? Did you ask the patient how he felt you could help him?*
> - *What did your management plan involve? Did you offer the patient help to stop drinking? Did you offer to change to a stronger dose or different proton pump inhibitor?*
> - *Did the patient seem happy with what you had suggested? If not did you take into account their beliefs when making these management decisions?*

Once again the exact nature of your management plan is not important. What is important is that you included the patient in the decision making process and gave them the option to decide what was best for them.

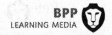

11. **When prescribing take steps to enhance concordance by exploring and responding to the patient's understanding of the treatment**

> - *If you had prescribed another proton pump inhibitor or a stronger dose of omeprazole for the patient did you explain how they work? Did you ask the patient how he thought they worked?*
> - *Did you explain that the stress and alcohol could cause excess levels of acid in the stomach and irritate the stomach lining? Did you explain that the proton pump inhibitor helps reduce the acid production and therefore helps counteract these effects?*
> - *If you were changing the dose did you explain why? If you were changing him to a different medication did you explain why also?*
> - *Did you explain to him how he should take the medication?*

12. **Specify the conditions and interval for follow up and review (safety net)**

> - *Did you offer the patient another appointment to see how they were getting on with cutting down on their drinking? Was this appointment in a reasonable time-frame, e.g. weeks as opposed to months?*
> - *Did you safety net and warn the patient that he should return if he had any red flag symptoms e.g. weight loss, haematemesis, black stools, appetite loss?*

13. **Confirm the patient's understanding**

> - *Did you actively take steps to ensure the patient had understood what you had said?*
> - *Did you ask him to summarise what you had said? Did the patient summarise the information correctly?*

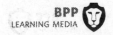

Notes

The patient was told to come across as quite intimidating and therefore the consultation could have gone wrong if you had not kept calm during the consultation. Although the patient may have been quite difficult to deal with, you should have not let his naturally assertive personality distract you. The important thing was to explore what he was concerned about, and if you did not do this you would have missed out on the fact he was worried about an ulcer as he had this previously. You would have also missed on the crucial fact that he is worried this is a sign he is drinking too much and he was told to only give you this information after a lot of pushing from yourself. Therefore, had you not taken steps to ask him about his work and personal life you would have not picked up on the clues he was going to give you about his drinking habit.

If the patient was not happy with your management plan, it may have been because you focussed too much on his drinking problem without exploring the reasons behind it. If you decided to immediately talk about the fact he should cut down on his drinking the patient would naturally become quite defensive. If this happened replay the consultation, this time exploring why he is drinking so much and what has happened recently to have caused this. If the patient reveals the information to you be sympathetic and empathise with how difficult the break up with his wife must be on him. If you do this the patient is more likely to be open to any suggestions you have about his drinking.

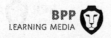

Mock Consultation 8

Doctor's brief

> Mr Tripolani, who is a patient of yours, has come to discuss his daughter Trisha. She is 19 years of age and is also a patient at your surgery. You had seen her about a week ago when she came to you to discuss the fact that she was depressed. Mr Tripolani is very upset today as he is worried about his daughter and wants you to tell him what was said when you saw Trisha a week ago. Trisha has told him that she had seen you but did not reveal what about.

You have 10 minutes to complete this task.

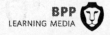

Use this space for your pre-consultation notes.

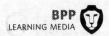

Mock Consultation 8

Patient's brief – *Do not read if you are playing the role of the doctor*

> You are Mr Tripolani, a widowed man with three children. Trisha is the youngest of your children and is also the only girl. As a result you have always been very over-protective of her, especially since her mother died five years ago. You have become increasingly worried because Trisha seems moody and withdrawn and you think she is depressed. She will not talk to you or her siblings about what is going on with her and this is concerning you. You would like her to speak to someone about how she is feeling.
>
> Your wife committed suicide five years ago and you had no idea at the time that she was feeling so low, as she too was very withdrawn. Subsequently, you are very worried that the same thing will happen to Trisha unless you deal with the matter. You are working at the moment and have no features of depression, although you are naturally very anxious about your daughter. You were aware that she saw her GP a week ago and want to know what was said. You are very angry initially as you feel that as her father, her GP should inform you about any problems she was having.
>
> Deep down you are aware that the GP is unable to inform you about what was said due to confidentiality reasons. However, unless the doctor specifically elicits the reasons as to why you are so concerned and empathises with you, you refuse to simply accept that he cannot tell you what Trisha has said. However, if the doctor is sympathetic to how you feel, you accept that he cannot tell you what has been said, but trust that he has Trisha's best interests at heart.

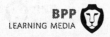

Mock Consultation 8

Information from the brief

Things you may have picked up from the brief are:

Mr Tripolani, who is a patient of yours, has come to discuss his daughter Trisha. She is 19 years of age and is also a patient at your surgery

This is telling you that you know both Mr Tripolani and his daughter, which may be relevant to how you deal with the matter. It may also be relevant to what he expects from you, especially if he sees you as a friend of the family. It is also telling you that he has come to discuss his daughter who is 19 years of age. This obviously will make it a difficult consultation as Trisha is an adult and entitled to confidentiality. It is also even more complicated by the fact that Mr Tripolani is also your patient and you also have a duty of care to him. Therefore you should be prepared for a difficult consultation.

You had seen her about a week ago when she came to you to discuss the fact that she was depressed

This may be giving us a clue as to what her father wishes to discuss with us. As she is suffering from depression, it is feasible to propose that her father has noticed her low moods too. However, we cannot assume this is the reason he is here.

Mr Tripolani is very upset today as he is worried about his daughter and wants you to tell him what was said when you saw Trisha a week ago

We are now aware that Mr Tripolani is very worried about his daughter. Why might this be? Is it due to the fact she seems depressed or is it another reason? How might this be affecting Mr Tripolani? What are his main concerns about Trisha? What does he think is going on with Trisha? These are questions we will need to address later. Also as we are told that Mr Tripolani is upset and worried, we will need to make sure we are sympathetic in our manner and appreciate his concerns.

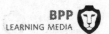

Trisha has told him that she had seen you but did not reveal what about

We are specifically told that Trisha has told him that she had seen us. Therefore we are allowed to say that Trisha did come to see us, although we will not be able to reveal the details of the consultation.

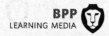

Mock Consultation 8

Suggested approach to the consultation by the doctor

1. Creating a safe environment for the patient

> - *Was the furniture appropriately placed so there were no obstacles between you and the patient?*
> - *The patient came in initially quite angry. How did you react to this? Did you remain seated even if the patient was standing? Or did you stand up as well which could be deemed as confrontational to the patient? Did you try to get the patient to sit down to diffuse the situation?*
> - *If the patient was shouting did you stay calm? Or did you also raise your voice?*
> - *What was your body language like? Did you become defensive when the patient was aggressive? Or did you pay particular attention to not be threatening yourself?*
> - *Did you empathise with the patient at the appropriate points?*

2. Introduction and opening statement

> - *Did you greet the patient using the name that was given in the brief?*
> - *The brief stated that you knew the patient and therefore you may not have introduced yourself. However, in view of the fact that you already knew the patient, did you make him feel comfortable by perhaps saying that it was nice to see him again?*
> - *Did you use an open question when asking the patient what had brought him to see you today?*

3. Encourage the patient's contribution at appropriate points in the consultation

> - *Did you take active steps to show the patient you were listening e.g. nodding your head, maintaining eye contact?*

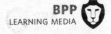

> - *Did you encourage the patient to continue if he paused or had difficulty revealing the information to you?*
> - *Did you show empathy if the patient seemed upset?*

e.g. *'I can understand this is upsetting for you to discuss. Please take your time.'*

4. **Respond to cues that lead to a deeper understanding of the problem**

> *The patient was obviously very angry/upset. Did you reflect that back to the patient?*

e.g. *'You seem very angry/upset today.'*

> - *When you reflected these feelings back did the patient explain why he felt that way?*
> - *Did you watch the patient carefully to look for non-verbal clues? Or were you distracted by his angry manner?*
> - *Did you listen to the patient without interrupting to be able to pick up on any hints he was giving you?*

e.g. *'I don't want the same thing to happen to her as happened to her mother.'*

> *Did you enquire more about what happened to her mother?*

5. **Elicit appropriate details to place the complaints in a social and psychosocial context**

> - *Did you ask Mr Tripolani how his worries about Trisha were affecting him? Did he then reveal to you that he was very worried about this matter?*
> - *Did you ask him how it was affecting the other members of the family? Did you ask him who else was at home with him and Trisha? Did you then realise that it was only himself and his children as his wife had passed away?*

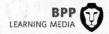

> - *Did you ask him if this was affecting his work?*
> - *Did you ask him how this was affecting his relationship with Trisha? What was their relationship like before this happened?*

6. **Explore the patient's health understanding**

> - *Did you ask Mr Tripolani what he felt was going on with Trisha?*
> - *Did you ask him what his main concern was with her behaviour? Did he then tell you about his wife's suicide and his concerns that she too, like Trisha, was very withdrawn before she took her own life?*
> - *Did you ask him what he was hoping would happen today? Was he hoping that you would tell him what Trisha had said? Or was he just more concerned that Trisha received the help that she needed?*

7. **Obtain sufficient information to include or exclude likely relevant significant conditions**
   As this case is about trying to sympathise with the patient and explain delicately that you cannot reveal confidentiality there is no need to take a history.

> *However, did you ask Mr Tripolani more about his mood and how he was coping? Did you ask him about his eating and sleeping patterns to ensure he was not also depressed?*

8. **Choose an appropriate physical or mental examination**
   This is not appropriate for this consultation. There was no need to examine the patient.

9. **Make a clinically appropriate working diagnosis / explain the diagnosis to the patient in appropriate language taking into account the patient's elicited beliefs**

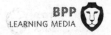

The 'diagnosis' in this case was really your explanation to the patient that you could not break confidentiality and the reasons why.

> • *Did you explain to Mr Tripolani why you were not allowed to break confidentiality? Did you do this in language he could understand?*
>
> • *When explaining that you could not break confidentiality, did you sympathise with how he must be feeling incorporating what he told you about his wife's suicide and his concerns over Trisha's mood? Or did you simply tell him that you could not reveal what Trisha had told you?*
>
> • *Did you ensure that you did not reveal any information that Trisha had told you she was depressed?*

10. **Make an appropriate management plan / involve the patient in significant management decisions**

> • *Did you ask Mr Tripolani how he felt you could help him? Did you ask him how he felt you could help Trisha?*
>
> • *Did you offer Mr Tripolani some support in coping with this difficult time? Or did you simply tell him that you could not break Trisha's confidentiality and leave it at that?*
>
> • *Did you suggest that perhaps he should try to talk to Trisha about his concerns?*
>
> • *If you did offer him some support did you give him a choice in the matter? What were those choices between? Did you offer him counselling? Did you offer him a follow up appointment to see how things were going?*
>
> • *Did you offer to see Trisha if she wanted to see you? Although you may already have a follow up appointment with her you were obviously not allowed to tell her father that. Therefore offering to see Trisha if she wanted to see you may have been a reasonable compromise. At least then her father would feel that you are trying to help and it negates the need for you to tell her father that you have already discussed Trisha's depression with her.*

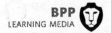

11. **When prescribing take steps to enhance concordance by exploring and responding to the patient's understanding of the treatment**

Unless you prescribed Mr Tripolani medication this is not relevant. As the brief stated that he was not depressed and had no features of depression there should have been no need to prescribe any medication.

12. **Specify the conditions and interval for follow up and review (safety net)**

> - *Did you offer Mr Tripolani a follow up appointment? Was this in a reasonable time frame?*
> - *Did you tell Mr Tripolani that if he has concerns over Trisha's safety or if he feels things are deteriorating he should let you know?*

13. **Confirm the patient's understanding**

> - *Did you actively take steps to ensure the patient had understood what you had said?*
> - *Did you ask him to summarise what you had said? Did the patient summarise the information correctly?*

Notes

This scenario was quite different to the others we have discussed and a lot of the points in the marking scheme were not relevant. This was mainly due to the nature of the presenting complaint and the fact that we could not really take a history, examine or come to a diagnosis. We were also not allowed to reveal any information about Trisha which also made the consultation even more difficult. The main point of the consultation was to sympathise with the patient, however maintaining your stance that you could not break confidentiality. In order to be able to truly sympathise with Mr Tripolani however, you needed to elicit the information about his wife's suicide and therefore you needed to specifically ask him what was concerning him about Trisha's behaviour.

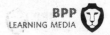

It was also important to be able to sympathise with how difficult it must be for him to see Trisha in this way, without informing him that she is depressed and had told you this last week. This can be quite difficult and therefore you should have not used the word 'depression' when describing Trisha, unless Mr Tripolani had mentioned he felt Trisha was depressed himself. Some of you may have felt that by telling Mr Tripolani to contact you if Trisha's mood deteriorates that this was implying you knew something already about her depression. This is not the case. Mr Tripolani has told you himself that he is worried about Trisha as she seems down and this is why he is concerned. You have not said anything about what Trisha had told you previously. Therefore, by informing him what to do if his suspicions worsen it does not mean that you have broken her confidentiality. However, at least by offering a safety-net you are making Mr Tripolani feel that he can come to you if things get worse and you are ensuring that Trisha is safe.

If the consultation did not go well you need to ask yourself why. Did you become quite defensive when the patient was angry and therefore was not sympathetic to how Mr Tripolani was feeling? Or perhaps you were too focussed on trying to tell him that you could not break confidentiality and did not explore his concerns? Although there was not much information to elicit from the actor's brief in this consultation, empathy and sensitivity were the key to a successful outcome.

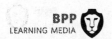

Mock Consultation 9

Doctor's brief

Mr Cooper is a 53-year-old man who has come to see you with erectile dysfunction.

You have 10 minutes to complete this task.

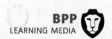

Use this space for your pre-consultation notes.

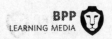

Mock Consultation 9

Patient's brief – *Do not read if you are playing the role of the doctor*

> You are Mr Cooper, a 53-year-old man who is having difficulty sustaining an erection.

Information unknown to the doctor

You were married for 25 years and never had any erectile difficulty before. You were divorced three years ago and have been single ever since. A few months ago you started dating a much younger woman who is 30 years of age. You get on very well with this woman and have a great relationship. Secretly however you are very anxious that if you do not perform well sexually she will leave you for a younger man. You are able to have an erection but are unable to sustain it due to the pressure you are putting on yourself. This in turn is making the situation worse as you are worried that you cannot satisfy her sexually and therefore are even more convinced that she will leave you.

You have no problems passing urine and have no symptoms of an enlarged prostate such as hesitancy, poor stream or dribbling. You are still having morning erections and can sustain an erection and achieve orgasm through masturbation. You are otherwise quite happy with life at the moment and have no other worries on your mind.

This is a very embarrassing subject for you and if the doctor gives you any idea that they feel uncomfortable talking about this subject you will not reveal your worries to them. However, if the doctor seems comfortable and can talk quite frankly to you regarding your sexual activity you become more relaxed. You do however, need a little encouragement from the doctor to talk about this problem, and show the doctor several times that you are reluctant to go on discussing this sensitive matter.

You will only reveal the information regarding your new relationship if the doctor specifically asks you about your partner, or asks you how your relationship is going.

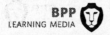

215

You are well aware of what is causing the erectile dysfunction, however as it is a sensitive subject you will only reveal it if the doctor asks you what you think may be causing it and has come across as sensitive.

You would like a prescription for Viagra today, however you are open to getting some psychosexual counselling to address your issues. You will only agree to do this however if the doctor has elicited your concerns.

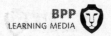

Mock Consultation 9

Information from brief

Things you may have picked up from the brief are:

Mr Cooper is a 53-year-old man that has come to see you with erectile dysfunction

This does not tell you much. However you are told his age which is therefore likely to have some relevance. You are also told his presenting complaint. You may have started to think about what issues could arise in a patient presenting with erectile dysfunction. As this is likely to have an impact on both him and his relationship you should be thinking about the psychosocial questions that you are likely to want to ask him. Obviously the impact his sexual difficulties is having on his relationship will be of great importance. It may also be an embarrassing problem so you should be thinking of ways to put the patient at ease. Therefore, although you are not given a large amount of information in the brief, you are given enough information to get you thinking about the questions you are likely to need to ask in advance.

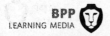

Mock Consultation 9

Suggested approach to the consultation by the doctor

1. Creating a safe environment for the patient

> - *Was the furniture appropriately placed so there were no obstacles between you and the patient?*
> - *As you had anticipated that this may be an embarrassing subject for the patient to talk about, did you place your chair a suitable distance away from the patient? Did the patient have to move their chair away because they felt uncomfortable?*
> - *Were you at an appropriate distance and angle to be able to see the patient's non-verbal expressions?*
> - *How were you seated? Was your body language appropriate? How did your body language make the patient feel? Did they feel comfortable?*
> - *Did you get embarrassed during the consultation thus making the patient more embarrassed? Did you lower your voice or mumble your words when mentioning words that you found embarrassing? Or did you remain clear throughout?*
> - *Did you empathise with the patient at the appropriate points?*

2. Introduction and opening statement

> - *Did you greet the patient using the name that was given in the brief?*
> - *Did you introduce who you were?*
> - *Did you use an open question when asking the patient what brought him to see you today?*

3. Encourage the patient's contribution at appropriate points in the consultation

> - *Did you take active steps to show the patient you were listening e.g. nodding your head, maintaining eye contact?*

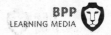

- *Did you pick up on the fact that the patient was having difficulty discussing this sensitive subject? Did you try to encourage the patient to reveal the information to you perhaps by acknowledging that you realise this must be a difficult topic for them to discuss?*
- *Did you encourage the patient to continue if he paused or had difficulty revealing the information to you?*
- *If the patient was initially reluctant to tell you what was worrying him, did you leave it at that or did you try to pursue the matter? If you pursued this further, did you do this appropriately and sensitively? Or did you directly keep asking him questions that you could see he was uncomfortable answering?*

4. **Respond to cues that lead to a deeper understanding of the problem**

Did you pick up that the patient was embarrassed and reflect this back to the patient?

e.g. *'You seem a little reluctant to discuss this.'*

- *Did you watch the patient carefully to look for non-verbal clues? Did you pick up on the fact that he was embarrassed from his mannerisms?*
- *Did you listen to the patient without interrupting to be able to pick up on any hints he was giving you?*
- *Did you pick up on the clue that he was dating a much younger woman?*
- *Did you pick up on the clue that this was a new relationship?*

5. **Elicit appropriate details to place the complaints in a social and psychosocial context**

- *Did you ask the patient about his current relationship e.g. how long they have been together and how things were going? If not, why not? This would be crucial to all erectile dysfunction cases but especially this scenario.*

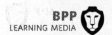

> - *Did you ask the patient how this problem was affecting his partner?*
> - *Did you ask the patient how this problem was affecting him?*
> - *Did you ask if his partner was supportive with his erectile dysfunction?*
> - *Did you ask the patient if he was having any problems in his relationship at the moment?*
> - *Did you ask the patient if he was having any other worries that could be affecting him e.g. work or other pressures? These outside influences could also have an effect on his sexual performance.*

6. Explore the patient's health understanding

> - *Did you ask the patient what he thought may be causing his erectile difficulties? Did he reveal to you that he felt it was the pressure he put on himself having a younger partner?*
> - *Did you ask the patient what his main worry about his erectile problems was? Did he reveal to you that he was worried his younger partner may leave him?*
> - *Did you ask the patient what he expected to happen today? Did he want medication? Did he want to investigate the problem further? Did he tell you that he wanted to try some Viagra?*

7. Obtain sufficient information to include or exclude likely relevant significant conditions

> - *Did you ask the patient what the exact problem he was having with his erections e.g. was it getting an erection or maintaining an erection?*
> - *Did you ask whether he could achieve erections under other circumstances e.g. during masturbation or early morning erections? If this was the case this would make an organic cause more unlikely.*
> - *Did you ask the relevant other questions to exclude any other pathology e.g. urinary symptoms, prostatic symptoms?*

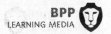

8. **Choose an appropriate physical or mental examination**

> *Did you realise that this was a psychological problem or did you offer to examine the patient later? There was no need to examine the patient in this case as it was clearly a psychological problem and there were no features in the history that suggested there was an organic cause for this. However, if you offered to examine the patient later you would not have lost marks.*

9. **Make a clinically appropriate working diagnosis / explain the diagnosis to the patient in appropriate language taking into account the patient's elicited beliefs**

> *   *Did you explain to the patient that you agreed with him that it may be the pressure he is putting on himself that is causing his erectile difficulty? If not, was that because you had not elicited what he thought was causing the problem?*
> *   *Did you explain to him clearly that this was unlikely to be a physical problem?*
> *   *Did you explain how stress and worry can affect an erection?*
> *   *Did you explain this in language the patient could understand?*
> *   *Were you sympathetic when explaining this to the patient? Did you empathise with how having a younger partner may make him feel self-conscious?*

10. **Make an appropriate management plan / involve the patient in significant management decisions**

> *   *Did you ask the patient if he had any thoughts on how you could help him?*
> *   *Even if he had mentioned Viagra did you mention his other choices e.g. other medications such as Cialis or psychosexual counselling?*
> *   *Did you ask the patient which option or options he would like to try?*

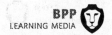

11. **When prescribing take steps to enhance concordance by exploring and responding to the patient's understanding of the treatment**

> - *If you prescribed Viagra did you explain to the patient how he should use it? If you did not know how to explain the usage of Viagra, did you improvise and perhaps tell the patient that at the end of your discussion you will give him a leaflet on exactly how to take it?*
> - *As the patient suggested Viagra did you ask him what he knew about it? Did you explain to him how Viagra works?*
> - *Did you explain to him what common side effects he may expect?*

12. **Specify the conditions and interval for follow up and review (safety net)**

> - *Did you offer the patient a follow up appointment to see if things were improving?*
> - *Did you offer him the opportunity to come back to see you at any time if things in his relationship should deteriorate or the medication did not work?*

13. **Confirm the patient's understanding**

> - *Did you actively take steps to ensure the patient had understood what you had said?*
> - *How did you do this? Did you actually ask the patient to summarise or repeat back to you what had been said?*
> - *Did the patient summarise the information correctly?*

Notes

This could have been a difficult consultation if this subject was one that you felt embarrassed about. If this was the case you may have shown the patient you were slightly uncomfortable discussing this, which may have meant that they became reluctant to give you the information. You may have come across as uncomfortable by your body language, or perhaps by being quiet or mumbling your

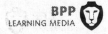

words when discussing the details around the patient's erections. You should have paid particular attention to this and ensured that you did not come across as unapproachable or reluctant to discuss this sensitive matter.

You were particularly not given a lot of information in the brief. Had you asked the necessary psychosocial questions about the relationship he was in and how it was all going you should have reasoned that the cause of his erectile dysfunction was likely to be psychological. However, if during your consultation you spent more time exploring all the possible organic causes of erectile dysfunction and you ended checking for diabetes or hypertension etc, you have missed the point entirely. This is either because you did not explore the psychosocial aspect of the presenting complaint or you missed the clues he gave you about his relationship with a younger woman altogether. However, had you mentioned to the patient that you would examine him later including checking his blood pressure after the discussion you would certainly have not lost marks for being thorough.

Following on from this some of you may have had different management plans and perhaps may have done blood tests to check for diabetes or a prostate specific antigen level. This would be perfectly acceptable as long as Viagra was also in the management plan, as this is what the patient actually wanted. Therefore had you not asked the patient what he had expected today or how he felt you could help you would have not picked up on this. Although it is all well and good ensuring that there is not a physical cause to his erectile dysfunction, this is not helping the patient immediately with his problem, and therefore you needed to offer him some sort of immediate help in your management plan.

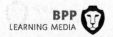

Mock Consultation 10

Doctor's brief

Mrs Rayner is a 73-year-old lady who has come to you as she is very upset. She had seen your colleague two days ago and was prescribed amoxicillin for a chest infection. She became very unwell after the antibiotics and developed a widespread rash with diarrhoea. She is allergic to penicillin and is very upset that she was given amoxicillin when this should be clearly in her records.

Additional information

Mrs Rayner is still symptomatic of having a chest infection, coughing up purulent sputum and having slight temperatures. She is not acutely short of breath today and there is no need to re-examine the patient. She did not have any lip or tongue swelling after taking the penicillin. Her rash and diarrhoea have also now settled. Her penicillin allergy is clearly documented in her records.

You have 10 minutes to complete this task.

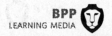

Use this space for your pre-consultation notes.

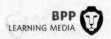

Mock Consultation 10

Patient's brief – *Do not read if you are playing the role of the doctor*

> You are Mrs Rayner, a 73-year-old lady, who was treated for a chest infection two days ago. You saw one of the GPs at the surgery at that time, who had prescribed you amoxicillin. You are allergic to penicillin and subsequently became very unwell and developed a widespread rash and diarrhoea after. You are very upset that you were given amoxicillin when you are penicillin-allergic. You have come to see one of the other GPs in the surgery as you did not want to see the doctor that made you unwell. You are still coughing large amounts of purulent sputum and are not feeling well in yourself. You are not short of breath however and are managing your normal daily activities without any problem.

Information unknown to the doctor

You were not aware at the time that amoxicillin was part of the penicillin family. You were not asked if you were allergic to anything and are appalled that you were given amoxicillin when your allergy to penicillin has been documented since you were a child. You are initially very angry when you see the GP and demand answers as to how this could happen.

Although you are very angry, you are truly very frightened. You live alone since your husband died and are feeling very lonely. You were extremely scared when you developed the rash and diarrhoea as you had no family or friends to help look after you. Being that unwell made you realise just how alone you are and you are very worried that you may become unwell again.

Although you are still coughing, you are reluctant to take any more antibiotics in case the same thing happens again. However, you do not reveal this information to the doctor, unless they specifically ask you how you feel about taking something else for your chest infection and explore your concerns.

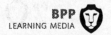

If the doctor is apologetic over what has happened and elicits your fears, you calm down and become open to the suggestions they give you. However, if they do not explore your personal life and the effect this is having on you, you remain very angry and demand to make a formal complaint.

If the doctor offers you a different antibiotic for your chest you are very reluctant and ask them several questions about if you will have the same side effect again. You only agree to take the antibiotic if the doctor explains to you why you need them and is sympathetic to how you feel.

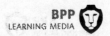

Mock Consultation 10

Information from the brief

Things you may have picked up from the brief are:

Mrs Rayner is a 73-year-old lady who has come to you today as she is very upset

The patient in front of you is an elderly patient and thus you should be thinking about what sort of psychosocial questions you may need to ask the patient. This may involve how they are coping at home or who is at home with them. You are also told that the patient is upset. Therefore, you need to prepare yourself to deal with a wide range of emotions from tears to anger.

She had seen your colleague two days ago and was prescribed amoxicillin for a chest infection. She became very unwell after the antibiotics and developed a widespread rash with diarrhoea

This sounds like an allergic reaction to the antibiotic. You should be thinking about how the patient is now and what effect these symptoms had on her. As it was your colleague that had seen her and given her the amoxicillin you may need to apologise on behalf of your colleague if a mistake was made. It should also prompt you to think about why she has come to see you when it was your colleague who was dealing with the matter.

She is allergic to penicillin and is very upset that she was given amoxicillin when this should be clearly in her records

This is telling you that the patient believes her symptoms were due to an allergic reaction. As she was given amoxicillin when she is allergic to penicillin this is a clinical error, and although your colleague may have been responsible it is your job to deal with it today. You should be prepared to be apologetic, even though the error was not your fault, and should not make excuses for your colleague.

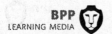

Additional information

This is telling you that the patient still has a chest infection. You should be thinking: why are you told that information? Is it because she still needs treatment for a chest infection?

You are told that she is not acutely short of breath, and did not have any life threatening symptoms with the allergic reaction. Therefore there is no medical emergency today. You are also told that her diarrhoea and rash have now settled. This information is reconfirming what you are told in the next sentence; that there is no need to re-examine the patient. Therefore you should not waste time doing so in the scenario.

At the end you are told that the penicillin allergy was clearly documented in her notes. As a result you can be certain that a mistake was made and the doctor was at fault.

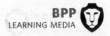

Mock Consultation 10

Suggested approach to the consultation by the doctor

1. Creating a safe environment for the patient

> - *You are told in the brief that the patient is upset. Therefore did you make sure that the furniture was appropriately placed? Was your chair sufficiently close enough to the patient to offer a supportive hand or tissue if needed? Did you make sure there was no other furniture or objects blocking your view of the patient?*
> - *Were you at an appropriate distance and angle to be able to see the patient's non-verbal expressions?*
> - *How were you seated? Was your body language appropriate? Did you become defensive when the patient was angry and upset? Or did you remain calm?*
> - *Did you keep a soft sympathetic tone when talking to the patient even when she was angry?*
> - *Did you empathise with the patient at the appropriate points?*

2. Introduction and opening statement

> - *Did you greet the patient using her name that was given in the brief?*
> - *Did you introduce who you were?*
> - *Did you comment on the fact that she had seen your colleague before?*
> - *Did you use an open question when asking the patient what brought her to see you today?*

3. Encourage the patient's contribution at appropriate points in the consultation

> - *Did you take active steps to show the patient you were listening e.g. nodding your head, maintaining eye contact?*

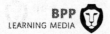

> • *Did you encourage the patient to continue if she paused or had difficulty revealing the information to you?*
> • *Did you show empathy if the patient found it difficult talking about certain things or was anxious to tell you how she felt?*

e.g. *'I understand this must be upsetting for you please take your time.'*

4. **Respond to cues that lead to a deeper understanding of the problem**

> • *Did you pick up that the patient was actually upset about a deeper issue other than her given the wrong antibiotics? Was there anything about her that made you think that this may be about something else?*
> • *Did you watch the patient carefully to look for any non-verbal clues?*
> • *Did you listen to the patient without interrupting to be able to pick up on any hints she was giving you, even when she was quite angry?*
> • *Did you pick up on her manner once she told you that she was at home alone? Did you pick up on the fact that she was actually quite fragile and worried?*

5. **Elicit appropriate details to place the complaints in a social and psychosocial context**

> • *As the patient was elderly and unwell did you ask her who was at home with her? Did she then reveal to you that she was alone?*
> • *Did you ask her how she was coping at home especially as she was alone?*
> • *Did you ask the patient if she had any friends or relatives nearby that she could rely on?*
> • *Did you sympathise with the fact that she was home alone and how frightening it must have been for her to have been so unwell?*

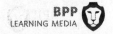

> • *Did you ask her how being so unwell affected her? What was she not able to do?*

6. **Explore the patient's health understanding**

> • *Did you ask the patient what she felt caused the rash and diarrhoea? Although the brief implies that she feels that it was due to an allergic reaction, did you ask her if she was worried it could represent anything else?*
> • *Did you ask her what her main concern about the rash and diarrhoea was? Did she reveal to you that she was very worried as she was home alone and is worried it may happen again?*
> • *Did you ask her what she expected to happen today? Did she want to make a formal complaint? Did she want to just make sure that the penicillin allergy was clearly on her records?*

7. **Obtain sufficient information to include or exclude likely relevant significant conditions**

   This point is not entirely relevant in this scenario because you are told about her symptoms in the brief. However you may have wished to verify the information in the brief, asking her if anything had changed with regards to her chest or if she was still coughing up phlegm. You may have also made sure that her rash and diarrhoea had truly settled.

> • *Did you simply ask her if she was still coughing up phlegm and having temperatures? Or did you ask her numerous questions about her cough, whether she was short of breath and ask her about other red flag symptoms?*
> • *Did you ask numerous questions about the rash and diarrhoea which had now settled wasting valuable time? Or did you simply ask her if these symptoms had settled?*

8. **Choose an appropriate physical or mental examination**

> • *Did you pay attention to the brief which stated that there was no need to examine the patient again?*

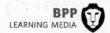

> • *If you did offer to examine the patient's chest, did you do it appropriately and mention that you would listen to her chest at the end of the consultation?*

9. **Make a clinically appropriate working diagnosis / explain the diagnosis to the patient in appropriate language taking into account the patient's elicited beliefs**

> • *Did you agree with the patient that her symptoms were representative of an allergic reaction? If not why not? Was it because you did not take the time to ask her what she felt was the cause of the diarrhoea and rash?*
> • *Did you explain to her that amoxicillin is a form of penicillin hence why she had an allergic reaction?*
> • *Did you also agree that an error had been made and she should not have been given amoxicillin as it is documented in her notes that she is penicillin-allergic?*
> • *Did you apologise for the error or did you make excuses as to why your colleague may have given her the medication? This would have not been appropriate.*
> • *Did you empathise with her in how frightening it must have been for her to have had this reaction when she was home alone with no family or friends nearby to rely on?*
> • *Did you explain to her that it still sounds like she has a chest infection and that as she had to stop the antibiotics it means that her chest infection has been left untreated?*

10. **Make an appropriate management plan / involve the patient in significant management decisions**

> • *Did you explain sympathetically to the patient that although she must be worried after the reaction she had the last time, she may need to still take another antibiotic as she still has a chest infection?*
> • *Did you explain to her that you can give her an antibiotic that is definitely not in the penicillin family and should not cause the adverse reaction she had before?*

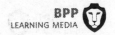

> - *Did you discuss her other options, for example giving her a delayed prescription of antibiotics she could use if she was no better or not having antibiotics at all?*
> - *Did you explain the potential risks and benefits of not taking the antibiotics or waiting until she got worse to take them?*
> - *Did you ask the patient how she feels about taking another antibiotic? Did you ask her what she would like to do?*

11. **When prescribing take steps to enhance concordance by exploring and responding to the patient's understanding of the treatment**

> - *If you prescribed an antibiotic e.g. erythromycin did you warn her about the common side effects? Did you ask her what she understood about antibiotics? If she did not know much did you explain how they worked?*
> - *Did you explain that she may still get some diarrhoea as this is common to all antibiotics and this does not mean she is allergic? If not, why didn't you? Did you feel this would worry the patient more? What do you think would happen to the patient if she suddenly had these side effects without you warning her?*
> - *Did you explain what she should do if she had any problems with the antibiotics? Did you explain to her how to take them? Or how long she needs to take them for?*

12. **Specify the conditions and interval for follow up and review (safety net)**

> - *Did you tell the patient that she must contact you immediately if her chest infection deteriorated and she developed an acute shortage of breath, had very high fevers or coughed up any blood?*
> - *Did you offer her a follow up appointment to make sure she was better?*
> - *Did you advise her to contact you if she had any side effects or problems with the antibiotics you had given her?*

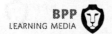

13. Confirm the patient's understanding

> - *Did you actively take steps to ensure the patient had understoodwhat you had said?*
> - *Did you ask her to summarise what you had said? Did the patient summarise the information correctly?*

Notes

The main points in this consultation were to be apologetic for the error and to not make excuses for what was clearly a significant event. However, at the same time you should not have let this distract you from what was a very frightening experience for an elderly patient. Therefore, if the consultation went wrong it is likely because you either made excuses for the error or did not appreciate the impact it had on the patient.

Some of you may have felt that you had no option in the management plan but to prescribe antibiotics, as the patient still had a chest infection. Therefore, you may have not given the patient a choice in how to manage her chest infection. Although you may feel it is in the patient's best interests to have antibiotics, you still need to give her a choice in the matter. This may have included having antibiotics immediately, having a delayed prescription that she should use if she felt no better or not having antibiotics at all. Obviously there is a risk that if she did not take the antibiotics she could become very unwell and you needed to have explained this to the patient. You should have explained why you felt she should have another course of antibiotics, taking into account how upsetting her previous experience was, but left the decision down to her. The patient was specifically told that she would accept the antibiotics if you explained to her why she needed them and was sympathetic to how worried she feels.

Similarly, some of you may have been reluctant to discuss the side effects of the antibiotics in case it worried her more. You would have been unlikely to have lost many marks for this in the exam as you are not being marked on your clinical management plan. However, you should have thought about the patient and how panicked she may get if she had a slightly loose motion thinking that the same thing could happen again.

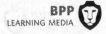

As a result it would have been better to warn the patient that she may have some diarrhoea, but this was to be expected. If you had explained how antibiotics work and the fact that they can kill the good bacteria in the bowel, the patient would have been likely to understand that this is a potential side effect she couldn't really avoid.

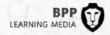

Chapter 4

The prioritisation exercise

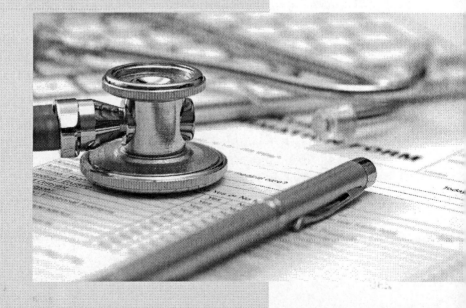

The prioritisation exercise

One of the most vital skills required of a good doctor, and particularly a General Practitioner, is the ability to prioritise tasks. General Practice is perceived by many to be less stressful than hospital medicine, providing a more favourable work/life balance. However, some days can be very busy, with the requirement for many tasks to be scheduled into a short period of time. You have probably found yourself in a similar situation as a junior doctor, perhaps for example after a busy day post-take. How do you decide what you need to do now, and what can you leave for later? How do you go about doing your jobs? Do you ask for help? Who do you approach for help?

This is what the Prioritisation Exercise of the selection process aims to assess. This chapter will explore the mark scheme used, approaches that can be taken to answer the exercises and ten exercises that can be completed to help ensure you are fully prepared. To ensure you make the most of the practical exercises in this chapter you can download blank answer sheets from www.bpp.com/freehealthresources.

> *The nature of general practice work involves the prioritisation of complex situations and tasks on a daily basis. These may, for example, be clinical, organisational, political or personal. This exercise gives a sense of the requirement for rational and logical thinking so that appropriate decision-making skills are developed and utilised when necessary.*
>
> Dr Dev Malhotra
> GP Trainer in Croydon VTS, London Deanery
> Partner in Brigstock Medical Practice

> *A reality of general practice is not knowing what the working day may bring. There may be doctor and staff illnesses/absences, shortage of appointments, personal crises and other emergencies that demand our attention – often all at once! The Prioritisation Exercise is an opportunity for candidates to demonstrate level-headedness in managing competing problems or issues.*
>
> Dr John Chan
> VTS Programme Director in the London Deanery
> GP Tutor for Croydon
> Partner in Eversley Medical Centre

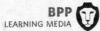

The format of the prioritisation exercise

The setting of the Prioritisation Exercise is similar to any other written assessment. You sit at individual desks until you are told to turn the page over. Most deaneries will initially ask you to open the paper, and read through the information provided for five minutes without being able to write anything. You will then have approximately 30 minutes to formulate your answers in the relevant boxes.

The exercise description you will be faced with consists of the following:

- A paragraph describing the setting and what your role is. This could be in primary or secondary care. So you may be the FY1 on ward cover in the evening on a busy medical ward. Or you may be the duty GP in a busy practice.
- This is followed by a list of five or six tasks that need to be completed, which will either be numbered (e.g. 1–6) or lettered (A–F). These could relate directly to the clinical aspects of patient care. For example, you may be asked to review a patient who is experiencing severe chest pain. Alternatively, they could involve something which is not directly related to patient care, such as an administrative task, or they could be something personal, for example you may have received a phone call that your spouse or child is ill.
- Also included will be a set of clear instructions asking you to rank the tasks, justify why you have ranked them in that order, and discuss the related issues around each of them. You will be given clear instructions on how to practically complete the exercise and it is important that you adhere to these as they will differ between Deaneries. For example to rank your tasks you may need to write your justifications in the order that you would complete the task. The time available to complete the whole exercise will be provided, as well as the time allowed at the start to read but not write anything.
- Finally, you will be asked to reflect on one aspect of the task. This is where you have to reflect upon what you have done, and discuss the points around this.

An example exercise is given for you to practise under timed conditions before you progress any further with this chapter. Possible answers will then be discussed as this chapter progresses.

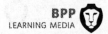

Example prioritisation exercise:
Scenario 1

You are the medical SHO covering the wards in a busy District General Hospital in the evening and have a number of jobs to do. The Registrar is busy in A&E seeing admissions, while the FY1 is on another ward.

Write the tasks in the order that you intend to rank them from 1 to 5, where 1 is the first task you would do, and 5 is the last. Write the letter of the task in the box provided. Justify your ranking and discuss any relevant issues relating to how you reached your decision. Write your answers within the box provided only.

At the start of the exercise you will be given five minutes to read the question, when you will not be allowed to write. Following this you will have 30 minutes to complete your answers in the boxes provided.

Tasks

A) A GP has called you to discuss a query about a drug you prescribed on a patient's discharge summary, as the patient is now unwell. The ward-clerk has put him on hold while he waits for you to get back to him.

B) A student nurse shouts across the ward asking you to bring the resuscitation trolley immediately.

C) The son and daughter of an elderly patient with disseminated bowel cancer arrive on the ward to discuss his 'Not For Resuscitation' status.

D) Your wife has left a message on your phone asking you to ring back as soon as possible.

E) Several drug charts are full and need to be re-written.

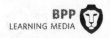

1. TASK
2. TASK
3. TASK
4. TASK
5. TASK
Reflection: What have you learnt from this exercise?

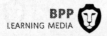

National Person Specification criteria assessed in the prioritisation exercise

During the Prioritisation Exercise you will be expected to demonstrate the following skills outlined in the Person Specification:

- Problem Solving and thinking around concepts [PS]
- Communication Skills [CS]
- Professional Integrity [PI]
- Coping with Pressure [CP]

These criteria relating to the Prioritisation Exercise are complex and can be further subdivided into sub-criteria which are explained in more detail below. You will be awarded marks based on each of these sub-criteria, and will be used to devise your final score. In order to excel in the Prioritisation Exercise, you must familiarise yourself with and understand how the NPS criteria relates to this part of the selection process.

Problem solving

Awareness of ambiguity

The amount of information that you are given is deliberately limited. If we look at Task A, there are plenty of questions one could raise, and plenty of information missing. For example what is the drug in question? Obviously, if it is diazepam or lithium, you would probably rush to the phone and find out what the dose is immediately. In contrast, if it is an aqueous cream or fybogel, you would probably deprioritise it.

The assessors want you to acknowledge that you may require further information. They want to see how you deal with this, and whether you consider all the possibilities, ranging from the best-case scenario (e.g. the GP wants to know the dose of laxatives for an elderly man with chronic constipation) to the worst-case scenario (e.g. this is an acutely psychotic patient who has possibly taken a benzodiazepine overdose). While acknowledging that you may need more information in some cases, you still have to use the limited information you have in the most effective way to formulate a plan of action.

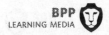

Thinking around issues

Generating workable solutions

The two sub-criteria above have very similar implications. It would be preferable to solve problems using the most direct, simple and straightforward methods. Going back to Scenario 1, in an ideal world all SHOs would be in a situation where ward-cover on-calls were quiet periods with senior colleagues always present to help if necessary. In such an ideal world, when dealing with Task A, you would take the phone-call, listen to what the GP wanted, go and find the discharge summary, then ring them back.

But the reality of on-call shifts is that there are almost always several challenging tasks to be completed simultaneously, often in difficult circumstances with limited time and no seniors around. A more realistic scenario is that while the ward-clerk is talking to you, your bleep has probably sounded five times, and two patients have deteriorated. So you cannot just pick up the phone and find the discharge summary as suggested. To solve problems in any difficult situation you will have to consider your individual circumstances, and improvise and innovate. To do this, you must think around the issue. Can you ring the GP back later? Can you delegate the task to your FY1, a nurse, or even the ward-clerk? Can you ask the ward-clerk to find the discharge summary while you speak to the GP?

This is what is meant by thinking laterally around the issue, and what it demonstrates is an adaptability that is essential for any medical career, especially General Practice. This will help you derive a solution that is feasible, and one that can practically work in your situation. There are usually several ways of dealing with a task, and you have to decide which will work in your scenario. The assessors want to determine if you are able to do this, and that is why the scenarios deliberately involve challenging circumstances.

Prioritising information and time

This is really the crux of the Prioritisation Exercise. You are faced with a number of difficult tasks, limited time in which to do them, and sometimes even limited resources and manpower. As mentioned earlier, you will often find yourself in this situation as a GP. Even as a trainee GP, you will certainly find it challenging

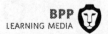

to prioritise seeing patients, checking blood results, dealing with repeat prescriptions and taking calls. As junior doctors, you have probably had similar experiences when on-call covering the wards on your own. This is why it is important to be able to decide which tasks need to be undertaken immediately and which tasks can wait. It is not possible to do everything simultaneously, and the only way to achieve this is through prioritisation. As a general rule, any task which involves immediate risk to patient safety should always be your first priority.

The Prioritisation Exercise also assesses your prioritisation of time by determining how well you cope with the time pressures during the actual assessment. Which is the very reason why you are deliberately given very little time to complete it. If you end up writing huge amounts for the first four tasks, and then hardly anything for the last two, you will score poorly on time management. It is obvious that if you were given an unlimited duration of time, you could consider how you would approach each of the tasks in far greater depth. However, this is not possible within the time allocated, and you will not be expected to discuss every single nuance relating to the tasks.

Communication skills

Sufficient communication with others

In both primary and secondary care, the multidisciplinary team (MDT) plays an instrumental role in ensuring the delivery of high quality patient care. A team can only function efficiently if there is clear and effective communication within it. Do you communicate enough with team members? How do you communicate with them? And do you communicate with everyone involved? In Task C, if you are unable to see the relatives immediately, do you talk to the nurse and explain why this is so? Do you talk to the relatives, and express empathy and consideration? In Task B, do you ask the nurse if they need help? Do you call your senior colleagues? If you go to that patient, you may have to leave other colleagues and patients you are currently with. Do you explain why you have to go, and why it is urgent for you to do so? It is important that you clearly state when, how, why and with whom you communicate. There are several ways to communicate – although much of your communication will be through talking to people, this is certainly

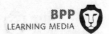

not the only way – e.g. putting out a cardiac-arrest call is also a way of communicating with the whole team. You need to clearly document all your communications, as the assessors will not assume anything.

Fluent written expression

The Prioritisation Exercise is the only task that assesses your written communication skills. What you write must be clear, coherent, structured and above all legible. Write neatly and check your grammar, punctuation and spelling. Make sure your answer flows, and does not sound disjointed. Write in prose and in full sentences – this way your answer will 'flow' well, and you can use the sentences to explain yourself properly. The advantages of this are that you can write quickly in short sentences, and you can easily distinguish one point from the next. However this can waste the limited space provided. Crossing outs, writing which spills out of the box, and answers not given in the format as instructed will create an impression that your written expression is not fluent.

Structuring your explanation

Your ability to structure the answer will be assessed by how organised your answers and intended actions are. You must demonstrate that you have thought your actions through in a way that is systematic and logical.

Persuasive varied expression

Some people are born writers, although most are not. Try to use a variety of words and expressions, even if you are describing the same concept. Avoid using the same words or sentences repeatedly. Place emphasis on important points, and deliberately less emphasis where it is not required. Try not to be repetitive, and if the same point has to be made repeatedly, use different words to describe it. This will make your answer sound more varied and persuasive, and will also maintain the assessor's interest in what you have written.

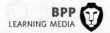

Use of sensitive language

Most of you will have been on the receiving end of insensitive remarks at some point in your medical careers, from patients, colleagues or both. If so, it will be easier for you to appreciate the importance of showing sensitivity and empathy. Even in very demanding situations, and when you are pushed for time, it is not difficult to show sensitivity. Going back to Task B – if the nurse wrongly asked for the resuscitation trolley and the patient was well, what would you do? Would you tell the nurse they requested you incorrectly, or would you ask them to explore their reasons for doing so? If their assessment was incorrect, would you hand them the resuscitation protocol, or would you offer them the protocol after explaining its importance?

Clear reflection

The Reflection question requires a different approach to the rest of the exercise, and merits a separate discussion in its own right which will be discussed later.

Professional integrity

1. Respect for others

2. Accepting of others

3. Balancing your own and others needs

These three sub-criteria are interlinked, and together constitute one of the most important aspects of the Prioritisation Exercise, namely teamwork. Emphasise the need to work with your colleagues in a considerate and constructive way. In Task B, it could be tempting to dismiss the student nurse as a non-qualified person who has limited expertise. But you need to accept that nurses will only exist if they undergo training, and thus accept student nurses as an integral part of the MDT. This alone is not enough – every member of the MDT, regardless of their seniority or role, deserves an equal amount of respect. Otherwise, team members will feel disillusioned and resentful, creating a dysfunctional team, which will ultimately harm patient care.

The GMC's *Good Medical Practice* guidelines state that doctors are obliged to 'Work with colleagues in the ways that best serve patients' interests'. However, the assessors are not looking for people who

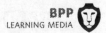

will sacrifice everything and anything they have for their colleagues. The reality is that healthcare professionals have their own needs. You have physical needs which you must recognise in order to avoid becoming overworked, as this may lead to a deterioration in performance to the extent that it could harm patient safety. You have emotional needs – if someone had a serious personal issue, such as a bereavement, they may be unable to perform normally. You also have professional needs, including the need to be trained by your seniors so that you can progress your career. However, it is important to recognise that all members of the MDT have such needs, and the diligent doctor will not only take this into account, but will also find practical ways of ensuring that everyone's needs are fulfilled as much as possible, including their own.

Positive approach to task

This is fairly self-explanatory. The assessors naturally want to avoid recruiting individuals whose main priority is to do as little work as possible, or who are cynical and disdainful of their colleagues and workplace. You must project yourself as someone who is optimistic, constructive and works hard to solve problems.

1. Comfortable with responsibility
2. Acting within professional boundaries

Being a doctor obviously carries huge responsibility. When you initiate or change a patient's management plan, you take responsibility for the benefits and adverse effects that result from it. Every time you sign a prescription, you take responsibility for every effect that drug has on the patient. This can be quite daunting when you first start working as a doctor, and it can be easy to 'pass the buck' and let someone else deal with a situation. However, the responsible doctor will make rational decisions which can be justified later if required. They will not deliberately walk away from responsibility, but rather embrace it as a challenge and as a unique privilege.

It is also imperative that you recognise your limitations, and the fact that you are not superhuman. Sometimes you will need help, and you can only do that if you are able to recognise your own limitations. One of the GMC's *Good Medical Practice* guidelines is to 'Recognise and work within the limits of your competence'.

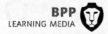

The MDT is vast, and there will always be someone who is able to help when you feel you are out of your depth. It is not enough to recognise when you need help, but you must also demonstrate that you are capable of using your colleagues effectively. In Task B, if you find that the patient is having a cardiac arrest, it would be naive to imagine that you can resuscitate the patient on your own. As an SHO, you will probably need manpower for physical assistance to undertake resuscitation, as you cannot effectively conduct chest compressions and ventilate a patient and read a monitor all by yourself. You will need help with clinical aspects from your seniors, such as your Registrar, who will have more experience in identifying arrythmias.

Coping with pressure

Acknowledging others' concerns

Empathy is important in medicine, not just towards your patients, but also towards your colleagues. In Task B, it may be easy to dismiss the concerns that the student nurse has because they are inexperienced and lack your level of clinical knowledge. The concerns that the patient's family have in Task C may be sidelined, because legally resuscitation decisions are medical. In contrast, an empathetic doctor will recognise that the student nurse's concerns need to be addressed both for their training needs to be fulfilled together with maintaining team cohesion. An empathetic doctor will also recognise the importance of considering the views of a patient's family in end-of-life decisions, and the deep-seated and long term effects this will have on the patient's relatives. This is what makes medicine unique through the need to combine interpersonal skills and empathy with scientific skills and clinical acumen.

Seeking help from others

There will be situations when you find yourself out of your depth in terms of knowledge and clinical skills. You are expected to recognise your limitations and ask for help when you need it. You may also need help if you experience a physically or emotionally demanding situation. Physical stresses may result from being overworked, and deprived of sleep or food. Emotional stresses may result from more personal problems, such as relationship issues.

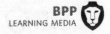

Maintaining perspective

As vague as this may sound initially, it relates to what is arguably the *raison d'être* of General Practice – holistic medicine. The GP is the doctor who can see the patient holistically, taking into consideration the vast plethora of biological, psychological and social circumstances influencing health and illness. Outside the realm of the patient, the GP is also the gatekeeper of the NHS, playing the key role of rationing the scarce resources allocated. This can only be achieved effectively if you have an understanding of healthcare systems, and how the NHS is managed. Maintaining a perspective relates to seeing the 'whole' picture and recognising that all aspects of patient care are interlinked.

Awareness of own needs

It is imperative that you recognise and address your own needs. To assess this specifically, there will almost always be a personal task. In Scenario 1, this is Task D. If you received a text from your spouse telling you to ring back urgently, how would you feel? What would your first priority be? Most people would be concerned that something untoward may have happened, and would want to ring back immediately. In this case, if you tried to ignore such a message and continued to work, it would probably affect your performance. This may even hinder patient safety. The assessors are not looking for masochistic individuals who have no personal attachments or emotions, but rather those who recognise their own needs and manage them appropriately.

Feasibility of solution

This relates to 'Workable solutions', and generating ideas that are not necessarily ideal, but can practically work in difficult circumstances.

How are you marked?

The assessors will reconvene at the end of the assessment day to score you on you have performed in the Prioritisation Exercise. They will grade how you have performed according to the NPS sub-criteria and mark your performance as follows:

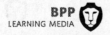

- No evidence
- Developmental need
- Mixed demonstration
- Sufficient demonstration
- Very good demonstration

Anecdotal evidence suggests that if you demonstrate 'no evidence' in more than two or three of the NPS sub-criteria, you will be automatically deemed unsuitable for GP training regardless of your other scores. If you are deemed unsuitable for GP training, it is very unlikely that you will even be placed on the 'Reserve List'. Breadth is more important than depth, so make sure you score reasonably well in all of the sub-criteria.

'Developmental need' and 'Mixed demonstration' indicate that you have demonstrated the NPS criteria, although not as well as the assessors would have liked. If you do attain the score necessary to enter GP training, then your Educational Supervisor may discuss the aspects in which you demonstrated a 'Developmental need' or a 'Mixed demonstration'.

'Sufficient demonstration' and 'Very good demonstrations' are self-explanatory.

The key to succeeding in the prioritisation exercise

Time management on the day

The biggest tip I would give for this task is to practise it beforehand under timed conditions. Most people ran out of time, as there is so much to cover.

Dr Gayathri Rabindra,
Trainee GP

The Prioritisation Exercise is by far the most time-pressured of the assessments you will face, and has been deliberately designed as such. Daily life in General Practice is time pressured, and patients have to be reviewed within ten minutes which is different to a hospital environment. There are fewer managers, and GP's are

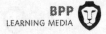

much more involved in devising the structure of their practice. This includes the practice as a whole, especially the allocation of resources such as time, money and manpower. Together with this GPs must structure their own day effectively. Time-management is hence an essential attribute required of a good GP, and perhaps that is why it features twice in the National Person Specification both within the criterion of 'Time prioritisation' and also 'Coping under pressure'.

Getting the right answer

> *There is no 'right' answer but what is sought is an approach that is well reasoned and justified – after all, we are all individuals and have our own priorities, but we need to translate these within the practice team context.*

Dr John Chan
VTS Programme Director in the London Deanery
GP Tutor for Croydon
Partner in Eversley Medical Centre

There are many ways in which you could tackle the Prioristisation Exercise, but it is imperative that you **justify** your answers. You must explain why you have ranked a particular task in that order, and provide clear reasons for doing so. Different people will have different priorities, but this does not necessarily mean that one is better than the other, or that one is right and the other is wrong. If it is clear that you have thought your answer through systematically, logically and in accordance with the GMC's *Good Medical Practice* guidelines and the NPS, it is likely that you will tick the right boxes.

However, it is important to note that there are always some obvious tasks which must be ranked higher than other less urgent tasks. Any clinical emergency where a patient's life is in immediate danger should always be your first priority. This is where some degree of clinical acumen is also necessary, as you must be able to recognise the patient who is acutely unwell. Most Prioritisation Exercises will include one such task which the assessors will expect you to prioritise above the other tasks.

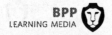

How to approach the exercise systematically

1. Read the description of the exercise carefully!

Use the allocated reading time at the beginning of the exercise to carefully read through the scenario, the tasks and the instructions provided. Familiarise yourself with the setting of the scenario (e.g. GP practice, hospital ward, A&E etc) and what your role is (e.g. SHO, FY1 etc), together with the time period of the scenario (e.g. you may have just started your shift or there may only be an hour to go until you finish). You should also begin to think about how you will prioritise the tasks during the allocated reading time and determine whether you must actually write your answers in the order that they are to be prioritised.

2. Limited time

Ensure that you have some form of watch to enable the efficient management of your time. You should aim to be in a position to begin writing as soon as the allocated reading time finishes. Considering that there are usually 5–6 tasks, you will have approximately 4–5 minutes to write about each task. It is important that you allocate each task a specific amount of time in this way, and move on to the next task in a disciplined manner once your allocated time runs out. This will ensure you cover all of the tasks, even if it is to a more limited extent than you may have ideally wanted to. Your time management skills will be deemed poor if it appears that you have written huge volumes on the first tasks, and then very little or nothing for the remaining tasks.

3. Rank the tasks – is anyone's life in danger?

It is useful to initially prioritise the tasks according to whether anyone's life is in danger, and how immediate this danger is. In a cardiac arrest situation, the patient's life is obviously in danger. With respect to urgency, the risk is immediate. The danger to life may not necessarily be related to a patient. If the task involves an angry violent person who has entered the hospital brandishing a knife there is also an immediate danger to life.

On the other hand, activities such as devising the on-call rota, or speaking to relatives are not associated with an immediate danger

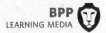

to life. It could be argued that they may indirectly endanger a patient's life if the rota is not organised properly.

However a patient who is confused, or wants to self discharge may well represent a danger to life through the cause or effect of his confusion. This is not as urgent as a cardiac arrest, but more urgent than organising the rota. On this basis, you can initially categorise tasks as follows:

- Definite immediate danger to life **(I)**
- Possible danger to life **(P)**
- Unlikely danger to life **(U)**

There are several other issues that must be considered when ranking the tasks and you could override the initial rankings you have devised on the basis of other issues.

Rather than trying to rank all the tasks immediately, it may be easier to decide on what tasks you would rank first and last. For example, there will often be a clinical emergency task which directly affects patient safety immediately which should be ranked first. Tasks which have minimal effects on the patient, yourself or the team could rank last. To rank something last does not mean that you do not think it is important. It merely signifies that it is relatively the least important of the tasks given.

4.   Limited information: best and worst case scenarios

You are provided with relatively little information for each task and you will almost certainly require further information to deal with the task efficiently. The uncertainty created by this lack of information should prompt you to consider the possibilities within the parameters of the information provided. For each task, discuss the worst-case scenario and the best-case scenario, explaining how you would deal with them. Do not make any assumptions, as this can lead to serious errors and misjudgements. If there is a vital piece of information missing that would help you in addressing the task, acknowledge that you do not have this, and hypothesise about the possibilities and how you intend to work around the problem. This demonstrates your awareness of the ambiguity around a problem, and the ability to think around an issue.

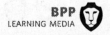

255

5. Who does each task affect?

The tasks can affect many people besides yourself and the patient. Think laterally. Consider all those around you including your team, your loved ones and those around the patient, including their relatives.

(a) **Patient**: As stated in the GMC *Good Medical Practice* guidelines the first duty of a doctor is to 'Make the care of your patient your first concern'. When thinking about the patient, also consider those around them, such as friends and relatives. Again, the GMC's *Good Medical Practice* clearly states the importance of giving consideration to patient's relatives.

(b) **Team:** Optimal care can only be provided to patients if the team functions efficiently. Hence, by assisting your team members you will indirectly be helping the patient. Decide which team members are being affected by the task before you intervene. Furthermore, working with colleagues effectively is also a professional duty as per the GMC *Good Medical Practice* guidance, and several of the NPS 'Coping with Pressure' criteria relate to teamwork. So any task that helps members of your team could rank high on this basis.

(c) **Yourself:** Remember that you are an integral part of the team, and it is vital for the team to function effectively. Hence it is important to look after yourself, and ensure that you not only address your work related needs, but also your professional career needs, your emotional needs, and your physical and health needs. A sense of professionalism and altruism can sometimes lead doctors to take on and do more work than they are physically capable of. However this can result in stress and disillusionment, and cause harm to your health. Apart from the negative impact on you personally, your performance as a doctor will also suffer, and could hinder your ability to provide optimal care for your patients.

There will almost certainly be a task relating to a personal or intimate issue that is likely to cause you varying degrees of distress and uncertainty. This will usually relate to a message or phone call. For example, from a close relative indicating that something untoward has happened to them or a message

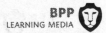

from your child's school asking you to ring back immediately. In some cases it may be something less serious such as getting your car back from the mechanic, or regarding arranging a holiday.

The assessors are not looking for masochistic individuals who plough on with their work at absolutely all costs. This is not only against the ethos of General Practice, the NHS and the GMC, but will also undoubtedly hinder teamwork and patient care. If you are distressed you may become distracted and make a serious error when treating a patient. Hence, it would be perfectly reasonable for you to rank such a task as a higher priority. This demonstrates various aspects of the Professional Integrity criteria, in particular the ability to balance the needs of yourself and others. On the other hand you may argue that although this task is important, you could deal with it later after the more urgent patient related tasks. This is an excellent example of the fact that there may be different approaches that can be taken. Different people with different characteristics and traits can react to the same thing in very different ways. Again, there is no correct answer, but make sure that you clearly explain and justify your order of prioritisation.

(d) **Other issues:** Clinical governance/Hospital/Practice/ Education/Ethics: there may be tasks that are related to systems rather then individual patients. These would usually relate to clinical governance topics such as audits and could probably rank lower. This does not mean that these issues are unimportant. Topics relating to management issues, audit, research and so on are important because they affect patient care and often the working conditions of medical staff.

However their effect is more long-term, and will usually take weeks, months or years to realise the benefits. Your scenario will usually be set in a busy GP practice, or hospital. On that basis it would be reasonable to acknowledge the importance of something like clinical governance, but to prioritise it below the tasks that relate more immediately to your patient, your team and yourself. This can be used to demonstrate your ability to think around issues as per the Problem Solving criteria of the NPS.

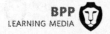

Hopefully this has illustrated that every task has varying degrees of impact on patient care eventually. Hence it is crucial that you think laterally about every task, and relate it to patient care even if the effect is indirect and over the longer term. Over the longer term all the tasks will lead to a chain of events, and this chain invariably finishes at the patient.

6. Utilising the MDT effectively

Consider how you will use your team, and how you will be of best use to them. There is no way you could tackle the tasks without full utilisation of your team. To do this well, you must be clear on the team members you will have at your disposal:

- **Doctors**: remember both your seniors (GPs, Registrars and Consultants), as well as your juniors.
- **Nurses**: this includes ward nurses, such as sisters, staff nurses and student nurses. In primary care there are practice nurses and Clinical Nurse Specialists, who specialise in one discipline, such as diabetes or cancer. There are also nurses who exclusively see patients in the community.
- **Healthcare assistants**
- **Palliative care/Macmillan Team:** there is often an end-of-life scenario, as these cover many aspects of care that could relate to various parts of the NPS, the GMC *Good Medical Practice* guidelines, as well as topics that are central to General Practice. These include ethics, communication skills, extensive MDT involvement and psycho-social issues. It also straddles primary, secondary and sometimes tertiary care.
- **Pharmacists**
- **Occupational therapists**
- **Physiotherapists**
- **Community psychiatry teams/Psychotherapists**
- **Social workers**
- **Patient Liaison and Advice Service (PALS)**: every hospital has its own PALS service. This is an NHS service available to everyone including patients, staff and the general public. The PALS team can provide support or advice on any issue relating to the trust, or refer people to someone who can. They can also take suggestions or comments to improve services.

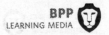

- **Administrative/clerical staff**: ward clerks in hospitals, and receptionists and practice managers in practices, can be very helpful and provide invaluable assistance with various tasks. Remember to think laterally, and beyond the clinical team if necessary.

Delegating tasks to appropriate team members is important to distribute the workload fairly, and to ensure that you do not become overloaded. This will help demonstrate the teamwork aspects of Professional Integrity, Problem Solving (in particular, generating workable solutions and prioritising time) and Coping Under Pressure (to devise a feasible solution using your resources such as the MDT).

However, remember the sub-criteria of Professional Integrity and Communication which relate to communication, sensitivity and respecting team members. Merely handing tasks over to colleagues will not cover this. State how you would communicate with your team.

The following is a list of buzzwords that may be helpful for this:

1. 'Talk to' colleagues
2. 'Ask', rather than tell!
3. 'Offer'
4. 'Suggest'
5. 'Reassure'
6. 'Bleep' or 'page',
7. 'Apologise' if necessary
8. 'Explain'

7. What, How, Who, Why, When

By now, you should have a good idea of how to approach each task in the scenario using a systematic and logical approach that considers the impact of each task on the patient and the people around them. Each task is a problem, and you need to provide a clear solution. It is easy to discuss the related issues and not specify exactly how you intend to solve the problem in the task.

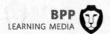

When structuring your response for each task you should initially determine exactly **what** needs to be done to solve the problem. Once you have done this, decide **how** you will achieve this and **who of your colleagues** from the MDT you will utilise. Decide **when** you will do the specified tasks, and above all justify **why** you have done this, relating it to the NPS criteria and the GMC *Good Medical Practice* guidelines.

8.   Follow-up, make sure it has been done

Once you have prioritised a task, decided what the solution is, and the methods, resources, and team members you will utilise to complete it, you need to make sure the task has been completed. Quite often you can identify a solution, initiate a plan of action, and later discover that the task has not been completed. The way to prevent this is by following up your plan and ensuring that is has been completed. You could even delegate the follow up to a team member and ask them to report back to you. The advantage of this approach is that if the delegated person is having any problems, you will find out immediately, and will have more time to take action. This will show that you are conscientious and comfortable with responsibility, which is a key part of Professional Integrity.

9.   Recognising limitations

As discussed, everyone has limitations in their knowledge and abilities. Recognising this is paramount for patient safety. This will usually be related to workload or clinical acumen. With respect to workload, you may find yourself physically overburdened with too many tasks, in which case you could delegate tasks to members of your MDT. With regards to clinical acumen, you may find yourself out of your depth when trying to make a diagnosis or compose a management plan. In which case someone with more experience and qualifications such as your Registrar or Consultant will be able to offer advice or assist you directly. You may have emotional limitations, as we have discussed with regards to the personal task. Recognising your limitations features in both the Professional Integrity and Coping with Pressure sub-criteria, which demonstrates its importance in the assessment process.

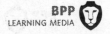

10. Comparing the tasks

Discussing the reasons why you have prioritised the tasks in the manner that you have is an integral part of scoring highly in the Prioritisation Exercise. Although all of the tasks are important, explaining how you have determined the order of prioritisation will be clearer if you discuss each task by comparing it to the others.

This approach will not only clearly justify the order of prioritisation, but will also encourage you to think about why you have ranked a task precisely where you have. This is what the prioritising time and information part of the Problem Solving criteria of the NPS evaluates.

11. Write, write and write!

Very few candidates are able to complete the Prioritisation Exercise with more than a minute or so to spare. There is a lot to write in a very short duration of time. However if you do find yourself with time and space to spare, then it is worth considering that the boxes have been made a certain size to reflect how much you are expected to write. If you think laterally around all of the issues relating to a task both directly and indirectly there are endless issues you could discuss. A word of caution though, it would be detrimental to continue writing if you have exhausted your ideas. If you start to 'waffle' and your discussion becomes incoherent or irrelevant, you may end up losing marks in the 'fluent written expression' and 'structuring explanation' subcriteria.

Summary of suggested approach
- Read the question carefully
- Rank the tasks based on patient safety
- Establish best and worst case scenarios
- Who each task affects
- Utilise the MDT effectively
- What, How, Who, Why, When
- Follow up
- Own limitations
- Comparing tasks

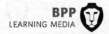

Reflection question

There will often be a question towards the end of the exercise which asks you to reflect on one aspect of the exercise, or the whole thing. But what is reflection? What does it mean to you? For many it is a vague term that means something philosophical where you have to think about something in depth. But more specifically, reflection is where you look back at something you have done and evaluate everything that happened. This involves thinking about what you did, what you did well, what you did badly, what you gained, and how that would impact on your actions and practice. People in all walks of life do this in some form or another – after losing a football match, you may go back to the dressing room, and discuss what went wrong, why it went wrong, and how you will improve your strategy, both collectively as a team and as individuals to prevent such a loss in the future.

In medicine for example, if you misdiagnose a serious condition, you would inevitably think about the incident at some point later, and devise a strategy to avoid it recurring. Indeed, learning medicine would be impossible without such a reflective process, and this is why the Royal College of General Practitioners has made it a requirement for GP trainees to maintain a 'Learning Log' of their reflective work, which is a prerequisite to progress through each year of training. Although no specific information has been released by the National Recruitment Office, anecdotal evidence suggests that the Reflection question carries as many marks as each of the other tasks within the Prioritisation Exercise.

Answering the reflection question

The importance of reflection in terms of the Prioritisation Exercise has already been clearly stated. The great thing about the Reflection question is that the questions you will be asked are usually very similar, and can include the following:

- What did you learn from this task?
- What did you learn about yourself from this task?
- What did you find difficult about this task?
- What did you find interesting about this task?

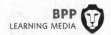

The answers to the Reflection question involve similar principles, and the following points can be used for the vast majority of questions.

Prioritisation is difficult

- Emphasise that the tasks are complex.
- There is a lack of information, creating uncertainty.
- There is a lack of time, both in the scenario, and even at your desk in the selection centre.
- The exercise does not consider the possibility of multitasking. In real life, you would often do more than one task simultaneously.
- Prioritisation becomes easier if you make a plan and identify key issues.

The task is interesting

- The tasks are very similar to the situation you often find yourself involved in day to day.
- All the tasks can eventually be related back to patient safety – some directly and immediately, others indirectly and in the longer term.
- The tasks are much easier to rank if you always put patient safety first.
- The MDT can be utilised in a variety of innovative and thoughtful ways to maximise team efficiency and subsequently patient care.

Learning about yourself

- You may have found that you naturally tend to put patient safety first.
- You may discover that you are able to think clearly and prioritise difficult tasks despite time pressures.
- You may realise the importance of personal issues, and how they may impact on patient care.

Which task is most difficult to rank?

- Often the task relating to personal issues (such as Task D) is most difficult to rank. The distress it causes may hinder your performance to the extent that patient safety is put at risk, in

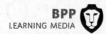

which case you could justifiably rank it higher. On the other hand, it could be argued that it is least related to patient care, in which case you could prioritise it last.

A personal perspective

There is advice that senior GPs and academics can give you. However some things are learned only through experience. The following advice has been collated from those who went through the process in recent years.

Before the day

Practise as much as you can

- Of the three parts to the Stage 3 assessment, this is by far the easiest to practise, as it can be done alone and your answers can be reviewed again later.
- Most of the questions are very similar, and the themes will certainly be common. If you have practised under timed conditions using the example exercises in this book you will become familiar with tackling exercises of this type.
- It is not only the logic and structure of your thinking that benefit from practice. The ability to write quickly in a limited space is a skill which is perfected only through practising under timed conditions.
- Time is the most important factor in this exercise. Practising will enable you to pace yourself properly. You will find that you are initially slow, but with practice you will naturally speed up.
- Together with the examples in this book try to formulate some of your own. Think of your last on-call, and five or six difficult tasks you had to do in a very short space of time.

Form a study group

- The best way to improve your answers is by asking your colleagues to read them. Do they understand what you have written? Do they think you have missed anything out? Can they read your writing? This is a task which requires extensive lateral thinking, and exposing yourself to other perspectives will be helpful.

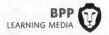

Sleep well the night before
- Many people stay up late the night before an exam in the hope that in the last few hours they will glean knowledge that will gain them the vital marks needed to scrape a pass. This assessment is different, as it is not your knowledge that is being tested primarily. It is your ability to apply knowledge in practical situations and think logically and systematically under pressure. You need to be able to think clearly and laterally on the day, and your mental faculties need to be in excellent shape.

On the day

Have at least two pens that you are comfortable with
- This task involves intense writing so having pens that you are comfortable writing with is important. Having a spare immediately to hand will ensure you don't waste valuable time switching pens.

Write legibly
- Although speed is important, it is easy to let your handwriting deteriorate unacceptably. This will reflect poorly on your ability to cope under pressure, your time management, and your written communication.

Make sure that your seat and table are comfortable
- Check that your furnishings do not have any problems as soon as you arrive at your desk. Wasting vital minutes in calling the invigilator once your time has begun will have a detrimental effect on your score.

Have a drink before you start
- Tea, coffee, lemonade, whatever suits you. Make sure you are energised and well hydrated. Most selection centres provide ample food and drink but it always wise to bring with you any food or drink you may feel you need.

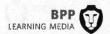

Start and finish exactly when you are instructed to

- Continuing to write after you have been told that the exercise has finished will risk disqualification and is not worth it.

Key points

If there is only one part of this chapter that you read and understand, make sure it is the following:

- **Justify** anything you write. Make sure you explain what you are doing in a logical, systematic and clear way.
- **Time** is very limited in this task, and probably the most decisive factor in how well you do. Pace yourself!
- **Remember the NPS competencies and GMC *Good Medical Practice* guidelines.** These form the basis of General Practice selection.

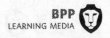

Worked example – Scenario 1

You are the medical SHO covering the wards in a busy District General Hospital in the evening and have a number of jobs that need to be done. The Registrar is busy in A&E seeing admissions, while the FY1 is on another ward. *Prioritise the tasks as follows:*

Write the tasks in the order that you intend to rank them from 1 to 5, where 1 is the first task you would do, and 5 is the last. Write the letter of the task in the box provided. Justify your ranking and discuss any relevant issues relating to how you reached your decision. Write your answers within the box provided only.

At the start of the exercise you will be given five minutes to read the question, when you will not be allowed to write. Following this you will have 20 minutes to complete your answers in the boxes provided.

(A) A GP has called you to discuss a query about a drug you prescribed on a patient's discharge-summary, as the patient is unwell. The ward-clerk has put him on hold while he waits for you to get back to him.

(B) A student nurse shouts across the ward asking you to bring the resuscitation trolley immediately.

(C) The son and daughter of an elderly patient with disseminated bowel cancer arrive on the ward to discuss his DNR status.

(D) Your wife has left a message on your phone asking you to ring back as soon as possible.

(E) Several drug charts are full and need to be re-written.

1. Read the information carefully

Read the information provided carefully and slowly. First make sure you know how many minutes you have to read through the question and how many you have to write. Here there are five tasks to be completed in 20 minutes, so you could decide that you will spend four minutes on each. As a medical SHO covering the

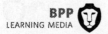

wards of a busy DGH in the evening, you will have your ward-based MDT to help you, including ward-clerks, nurses, an FY1 and a Registrar. The Consultant may not be present, although he or she will be contactable by phone.

2. Rank the tasks – risk to life

Try to do this mentally within your allocated 'reading time' using the system previously discussed:

- Definite immediate danger to life (I)
- Possible danger to life (P)
- Unlikely/no danger to life (U)

Task A

A GP has called you to discuss a query about a drug you prescribed on a patient's discharge-summary, as the patient is unwell. The ward-clerk has put him on hold while he waits for you to get back to him.

There is no immediate danger to life, because the GP would have called an ambulance if there was. There is a small possibility that the GP may be calling regarding an aspect of the drug which is pivotal to patient safety. If the GP suspects an internal hemorrhage and the patient is on warfarin, or is drowsy following the prescribing of benzodiazepine, there may be a danger to life. However it is unlikely that the GP would be waiting for you on the phone if this was the case, and even if it was, the GP is a qualified doctor who is at the scene and able to assess the patient and bring him to hospital if needed. Hence we can categorise this task as P.

Task B

A student nurse shouts across the ward asking you to bring the resuscitation trolley immediately.

This should immediately stand out. If someone is urgently asking for the resuscitation trolley, there is a strong possibility that they need it to resuscitate someone. Although the nurse may need the trolley for a totally unrelated purpose, there is a good possibility of an immediate danger to the patient's life, so this task can be categorised as I.

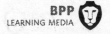

Task C

The son and daughter of an elderly patient with disseminated bowel cancer arrive on the ward to discuss his DNR status.

This is an important task for a number of reasons that we will discuss later. However there is clearly no danger to anyone's life. So this task should be categorised as U. This should not undermine its importance; all this means is that this task does not need to be addressed as urgently as a task where someone's life is in immediate danger.

Task D

Your wife has left a message on your phone asking you to ring back as soon as possible.

This is the personal task. As discussed previously, you could rank it highly arguing that it would adversely affect your performance to the extent that you may end up putting patient's lives at risk. However you could also argue that it has no bearing on patient's lives, is unrelated to patient care in any way, and could wait. It really depends on what you are like as an individual, and how you deal with such things on a personal level. The key here is to ensure that you fully justify your answer as to why you have ranked the task in the way that you have, for example you may be expecting news regarding your terminally ill father. You could justify categorising it as P, because the distress caused to you may result in your performance deteriorating. In contrast, if you feel you are 'thick-skinned' and can cope with it, you could categorise it as U on the basis that you would be able to continue with your work and call your wife after your shift finishes. Remember that this categorisation approach is purely to help you rank the tasks, so you can manipulate it to your benefit. For the purposes of this worked example this task can be categorised as a P/U.

Task E

Several drug charts are full and need to be re-written.

It is difficult to imagine how not completing this task immediately would put anyone's life in immediate danger. Even if a patient needs a drug administered immediately, it can be given as long

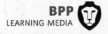

as it has been prescribed. Many drug charts have a miscellaneous section at the back where this can be documented. This task can be categorised as a U.

Based on this discussion of danger to life the tasks can be initially ranked in the following order:

Task A)   P   Rank 2nd
Task B)   I   Rank 1st
Task C)   U   Rank 4th or 5th
Task D)   P/U   Rank 3rd
Task E)   U   Rank 4th or 5th

We can now work through each task separately using the suggested approach.

Task B
A student nurse shouts across the ward asking you to bring the resuscitation trolley immediately.

Limited information – best and worst case scenarios
As discussed, the information provided to you is limited. First and foremost, you do not know who the patient is, and what their clinical situation is. They may have a terminal disease, and may be 'Not for Resuscitation'. On the other hand the patient may have stopped breathing and be lying unresponsive. It is possible that the nurse is actually asking for the resuscitation trolley for a different reason. They may need to refill its equipment, or they may want to familiarise with it for educational reasons.

Who does it affect?
(a) Patient: This task has potentially the most serious and direct impact on patient safety.
(b) Team: The student nurse is the first person affected by this. Other nurses on the ward may also be affected. There is no suggestion of any other team members being present on the ward.

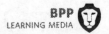

(c) Yourself: It will obviously be stressful and difficult for you if the patient is acutely unwell, and it will also affect the way you deal with the other tasks.

(d) Other issues: Clinical governance/Hospital/Practice/ Education/Ethical: there are various educational issues which may arise from this situation. If the patient is having a cardiac arrest, the student nurse should have put out a cardiac arrest call, or if she did not know how to do this she could have called a senior colleague. If the patient was not acutely unwell, it could be argued that her reaction was alarming and disproportionate. These are all learning needs which a student doctor or nurse may quite legitimately have. The GMC's *Good Medical Practice* guidelines state clearly that the teaching and training of colleagues is a professional responsibility. Although this is not the immediate priority when on-call, it is still vitally important because the student nurse has their own professional and educational needs.

Using the MDT

Think about the main issue to start off with. There is a possibility of a cardiac arrest situation, and that is what you need to deal with first. The only way you can determine this is by assessing the patient. You could be in the middle of another task at this point which you may need to handover very quickly to a junior colleague or a nurse. If the patient is found to be in arrest, you need to put out a crash call, which demonstrates that you recognise your limitations and that you cannot resuscitate a patient single-handedly. If your seniors are nearby, then you could call them and start resuscitation. If they are not around, you would have to start resuscitating the patient utilising the staff you have around you – which in this case will be the nurses on the ward. This demonstrates that you have devised a feasible solution under limited time, and also that you can use your team effectively. You should also make sure that the patient has not already had a 'Not For Resuscitation' form completed. Once the resuscitation team has arrived, you could even leave and hand over to them if they were sufficiently staffed and they were satisfied they could cope without you.

Alternatively, it could well be a false alarm, and there may be no need for a cardiac arrest call, or any immediate medical intervention. However, there are significant issues still to be dealt with. Remember

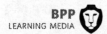

that the nurse is a trainee, and has educational needs. Teaching and training colleagues is your responsibility as much as anyone else's, and the recognition and management of acutely unwell patients may be a learning need for them. You could offer to help them in this, and perhaps organise a teaching session, or arrange one through the ward-sister.

Follow-up

Most tasks require follow-up to ensure that they are completed. However a cardiac arrest, or indeed any acute clinical situation requires immediate action.

If the patient is unwell but not as acutely unwell as thought initially, you could implement management, and reassure the student nurse that they should feel free to bleep you if later if they feel the patient has deteriorated or has any other concerns – this demonstrates your communication skills. You could also commend them for demonstrating concern and trying to manage an acutely unwell patient, which would demonstrate good teamwork skills.

Recognising limitations

As discussed with regards to the MDT, this may be an acute situation warranting senior intervention including the cardiac arrest team. Therein you recognise that you cannot manage this situation effectively on your own. Other than this, by delegating to your ward-clerk, nurse or FY1 while you are involved in resuscitation, you demonstrate insight that you cannot manage the acute situation and the other jobs simultaneously.

Comparing the tasks

This is easy for the task you rank first. You need to provide the reasons discussed above, and explain how the immediate danger to the patient's life is more important than any of the other tasks.

Task A

A GP has called you to discuss a query about a drug you prescribed on a patient's discharge summary, as the patient is now unwell. The ward-clerk has put him on hold while he waits for you to get back to him.

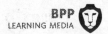

Limited information – best and worst case scenarios

Several questions arise when considering this task. First, how 'unwell' is the patient? Is his airway, breathing or circulation compromised? The possibilities are endless, and this may be a patient with a history of depression who has been found drowsy, and the discharge summary may be crumpled and ineligible. As mentioned before, the patient may have had an internal bleed while on warfarin. These are the worst case scenarios. However, it may be something much less serious – the patient may have a migraine, and the GP may want to know whether the paracetamol and antiemetic you prescribed in the hospital worked for this. This is obviously serious, as the patient may be in agonising pain. However, it is less serious than the other possibilities mentioned.

Who does it affect?

(a) Patient: The patient has been or will be taking the drug, and will derive benefit or harm accordingly.
(b) Team: The GP is affected because his management of the patient depends on this vital piece of information. He has to wait for you, which is probably holding up his work. The ward-clerk who is keeping him on hold is also affected, as she may have stopped some of her other jobs to do this.
(c) Yourself: You are affected because you have to find the most efficient way of finding the discharge summary and talking to the GP while managing your ward tasks simultaneously. You may feel pressured because a senior colleague is waiting for you on the phone.
(d) Other issues: Why has the GP had to call you at this moment? It is possible that the discharge summary did not provide a vital piece of information? Or are the discharge summaries not sufficiently clear or comprehensive? All of these issues relate to a system defect, and you could try to solve this by recording the problem as a significant event, and fill in a Significant Event Analysis form.

Using the MDT

The GP has called you for something that is obviously important to them. You need to demonstrate respect for a fellow team member and appreciate that they are waiting for you. This will illustrate your professional integrity. To reinforce your communication skills,

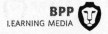

speak to them courteously and as soon as possible within the circumstances. The ward-clerk is keeping them on hold to make life easier for you, so thank her for her patience. You could also delegate the task to them depending on what the query is. For example, if the GP was missing part of the discharge summary, the ward-clerk could very easily find another copy and fax it over to the GP. After speaking to the GP, you could also delegate the task to your FY1 if they are able to do it. However remember that you must do it in a courteous way by politely requesting him to do so, and providing reassurance that they could bleep you if necessary. This will illustrate your ability to think around a problem, and also to find a feasible solution using the resources provided.

Follow-up

If you have delegated any tasks then it is your responsibility to ensure that they are completed. If you are faxing or sending something to the GP, it may be prudent to ring them later to confirm receipt. This demonstrates conscientiousness which relates to professional integrity.

Comparing the tasks

As this task has ranked below Task B you need to justify why. Your first argument could be that the patient is being seen by a fellow doctor who is more qualified and experienced than yourself. If the patient was acutely unwell the GP would have taken them to hospital immediately.

This task ranks above the other remaining task because there may be factors that could affect patient safety in the short-term. Your relationship with the GP and ward-clerk is also at stake, as they may become annoyed if left on-hold for too long. Again this demonstrates how important teamwork is to you.

Task D

Your wife has left a message on your phone asking you to ring back as soon as possible.

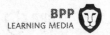

Limited information – best and worst case scenarios

This is a very realistic scenario. At some point in your life you will have probably received a message from a loved one which has caused alarm due to limited information provided. You would naturally think of the worst case scenario first. Has your partner been involved in an accident? Are they ill?

On the other hand, you may know that your partner is in a place of safety surrounded by people who would be able to help them if needed. It also depends on the context – you may know that your partner calls you every day to discuss trivial matters, in which case this wouldn't surprise you.

Who does it affect?

(a) Patient: Although not directly related to patient care, this task has the potential to affect you significantly. If you are severely distressed by this, you may not think clearly and become distracted, which would impair your decision making skills and possibly put patient safety at risk. Mistakes which tend to occur as a result of poor concentration often involve prescribing, a classical example being penicillin being prescribed to a patient who is allergic to it.

(b) Team: If you are distressed to such an extent that you cannot function properly, your team will also be affected.

(c) Yourself: As discussed above, the personal task affects you primarily. You may be very distressed, and your emotional needs may need to be addressed with empathy and consideration.

(d) Other issues: Medical staffing and Management: If you have to leave, it would be considerate to liaise with the hospital management and your colleagues to arrange cover in your absence. This is an excellent example of how you may balance your own needs with others in the team, as per the Professional Integrity criteria of the NPS.

Using the MDT

Despite the uniquely personal nature of the task, there are many ways in which you could utilise the team to your advantage. You could find out why your partner left the message for you by ringing her back immediately, which could be done very quickly. In the meantime you could delegate your work temporarily to

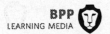

your FY1. However remember that they may also be busy with tasks. To maintain rapport with them, explain the situation and thank them for their co-operation.

You could even delegate the discussion with your partner to someone else. If you are in the middle of seeing a patient, you could enlist the help of the ward clerk. You could politely ask them if they would be happy to call your partner back to find out the reason for their message. Remember basic courtesies, including thanking them for their assistance and explaining the need to delegate (e.g. you may be in the middle of a sterile procedure). This course of action would also be very quick, to the extent that you do not even have to stop your current task, and would also demonstrate that you can think around problems and work effectively with your team, all important criteria in the NPS.

Follow-up

If you delegate work to your FY1, remember to follow them up as well, and find out how they have been coping. This shows your sense of responsibility. If you delegated it to your ward-clerk, then you will obviously follow it up because of the anxiety you have about your partner.

Recognising limitations

Most of the tasks relate to professional and logistical limitations. However, this relates more to emotional limitations. Recognising that you are human and have affinity for your loved ones is important for your own well being.

Comparing the tasks

You could rank this below Tasks B and A as it is not an immediate life-threatening emergency. It ranks above the others because of three reasons. First, the effect on you could hinder your performance and compromise patient safety. Second, it can be done very quickly – a phone call to your partner may only last one or two minutes. Third, you could argue that your own emotional needs are very important.

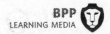

Task C

The son and daughter of an elderly patient with disseminated bowel cancer arrive on the ward to discuss his DNR status.

Limited information

There is a good chance that end of life issues will feature at some point in the Stage 3 assessment. Anyone who has worked in geriatrics or palliative care will testify that even with extensive information, these issues raise several possibilities and could be the source of extensive debates with a wide variety of opinions.

You would first want to determine how terminal the patient's situation is, and the prognostic time frame. If the patient is conscious, able to converse coherently and is competent, you may not be able to discuss even the most cursory of details with relatives without their consent. This would restrict your conversation with them, although you could show huge empathy and provide psychosocial support without compromising confidentiality. On the other hand, this may be a patient who is almost vegetative, and completely dependent on life support equipment. In this case, the family may be able to provide vital information on how far the patient would have wanted to progress with treatment in such a situation, and whether or not they would want to be resuscitated. The patient may have had specific wishes relating to culture or religion of which only their children are aware.

As doctors it is imperative that we respect patient autonomy, and establishing the patient's wishes would assist this. The GMC *Good Medical Practice* guidelines also recommend that doctors consider the views of family members when appropriate.

Who does it affect?

(a) Patient: As long as the patient is competent, they will decide the extent of their family's involvement. If they are not competent, the knowledge that the family have about the patient's wishes may be pivotal when deciding how to manage them, and how aggressive to be with their treatment. However the relatives are also under immense physical and emotional stress, and need to be treated with empathy and sensitivity.

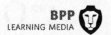

(b) Team: Organising high quality end of life care requires the involvement of various members of the MDT, and extensive input and flexibility. Remember that this is also emotionally taxing, and consider this when liaising with palliative or elderly care teams.

(c) Yourself: Talking to the son and daughter is not something that can be rushed and will take a significant amount of your time.

(d) Other issues: Ethics: End of life decisions, particularly those relating to resuscitation are an ethical minefield. Different people will have different views on how far treatment should go. Some will be argue that it is ethically wrong to not utilise the full armoury of medical expertise and resources. Others will argue that it is unethical to put patients through the associated indignity and pain. These are both valid arguments, and any answer that is well-justified, while maintaining respect and consideration for both sides of the argument is likely to score highly. Remember that 'acceptance' of your colleagues is part of the NPS, and try to avoid viewpoints that are extreme and representative of only one side of the argument.

Using the MDT

As always, start at the beginning. You are told by the nurses that the son and daughter of the patient have just arrived. There are a number of options you have available to you. If you have other more pressing tasks to do, you could politely ask them to wait in a patient's room, and perhaps even offer a cup of tea, or some other gesture of courtesy. You could also delegate this task to a ward nurse, saving you the time it takes to get to the ward. On the other hand, a ward-sister could start discussions with the son and daughter about what the main issues are, so that the 'groundwork' is done by the time you arrive.

You may want to involve the palliative care team in the discussions, especially if they have been involved in the care of the patient. They could help reassure the relatives that they would still continue to care for the patient, and emphasise that 'Not For Resuscitation' does not necessarily equate with the withdrawal of all treatment. They could also explain how they will try to make the patient's terminal stages as comfortable as possible both for the patient and the relatives.

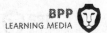

Follow-up, make sure it's been done

If you are participating in the discussions with the family, then you do not need to follow-up, as you will be present. However, if you delegate the task to a ward-sister then it would be prudent to make sure that the discussion has taken place. If you ask them to wait for you, you may ring the ward to find out how the son and daughter are, and make sure that they are comfortable. If you have delegated any ward tasks to the FY1 while you are in the meeting, you may want to bleep them at some point for an update.

Recognising limitations

The issues requiring discussion may be new to you, and you may need a senior doctor or a specialist cancer nurse to help you. The other wards may be far too busy for you to attend to the son and daughter, which is a limitation related to workload and time.

Comparing the tasks

You could justify ranking this below Tasks A, D and B because this task poses no immediate threat to life, and requires time to deal with properly. It could rank above Task E because it involves significant ethical issues, as well as relatives who require empathy and sensitivity.

Task E

Several drug charts are full and need to be re-written.

Limited information

Although this task has a narrower focus than the others, there is still vital information missing that could be decisive in where you rank it. There may be three or four drug charts for patients admitted due to social reasons who are relatively stable and awaiting placement. On the other hand there may be ten or 15 drug charts for patients who are acutely unwell, and are on medication vital for the maintenance of their basic physiology. Good examples of this include patients with upper-gastrointestinal bleeding who require blood and an intravenous proton-pump inhibitor, or patients with sepsis on powerful intravenous antibiotics.

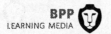

Who does it affect?

(a) Patient: As above.

(b) Team: Nurses are most directly affected by full drug charts, as they have to record the administration of the drug every time it is administered. Different hospitals have different policies. Some have drug charts with a section for drugs prescribed whose administration cannot be documented immediately. Some nurses will argue that it is perfectly legitimate to give medications that are clearly prescribed.

(c) Yourself: The nurses will continue bleeping you until you rewrite the charts – which is understandable from their perspective.

(d) Other issues: Hospital policy: As discussed above, every hospital has its own policy on dealing with 'full' drug charts. Some allow pharmacists to rewrite drug charts. In the longer term you could propose a policy whereby all teams check their drug charts and rewrite those which will be full by the weekend.

Using the MDT

There are several members of the MDT who could assist you in this task. If you are very busy, you could ask your FY1 to re-write the charts. Courtesy, explaining the situation, and reassurance that they can bleep you if needed, are all vital to maintain team cohesion and consideration for others. As discussed above, the pharmacists may be able to help. If the drug charts are urgent, and you are dealing with something more important on another ward, you could negotiate with the nurses, explaining why you cannot attend the ward immediately, and arrange for the charts to be brought to you by a nurse or a porter. Or you could compromise whereby the nurse collates all of the urgent drug charts for you to do immediately and return later to complete the others.

Follow-up, make sure it's been done

If you have delegated this to a pharmacist or FY1, check that they have done it, while expressing your appreciation for their help.

Recognising limitations

Other than time limitations, there may be limitations to your knowledge of drugs and pharmacology, and you may need to consult with a senior or a pharmacist.

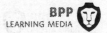

Comparing the tasks

The fact that this task is ranked last does not render it unimportant. The prioritisation merely indicates which tasks should be done immediately and which can be left until later. You could argue that it is unlikely that full drug charts will cause an immediate risk to patient safety, largely due to the pragmatism and astuteness of nurses who may continue administering the drugs and document it elsewhere. It is also a time-consuming task.

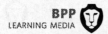

Suggested Answer for Scenario 1

To aid understanding each part of the example answers have been annotated in bold to illustrate how they relate back to the NPS.

- Problem Solving and thinking around concepts [PS]
- Communication Skills [CS]
- Professional Integrity [PI]
- Coping with Pressure [CP]

---

(1) TASK B

This is my first priority because of the following reasons:

The student nurse is inexperienced. The patient may **[PS – saying 'may' signifies uncertainty]** be having a cardiac arrest, and the student nurse may be unaware of the procedure in place to put out a crash-call. I would quickly **[CP, PS – you recognise the need to do it quickly, in view of the time pressure and the clinical urgency]** assess the patient then put out a crash call if necessary **[PS]**. If I was the most senior doctor present, I would start resuscitation **[PI – you have taken responsibility]**, and hand over to the cardiac arrest team **[PI, CP – you recognise your limitations and have involved the team appropriately]** on their arrival. I would only leave if and after the crash team have the situation under control and were happy to continue without me **[PI, CP]**.

However I also appreciate that this may be a false alarm **[PS]**. The student nurse may need the resuscitation trolley for an altogether different purpose **[PS]**, or may have overestimated the deterioration of the patient. First, I would comfort the student nurse **[CS, PI – this demonstrates empathy and consideration for your colleague]**, and then offer constructively to teach her personally about resuscitation and cardiac arrests. In addition to this, I would reassure **[CS, PI]** her that she could feel free to bleep me if she was concerned about the patient.

 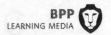

(2) TASK A

This task ranks below Task B because there appears **[PS]** to be no immediate risk to patient safety, despite the limited information about the nature of the patient's illness. Moreover, there is already a qualified doctor with the patient who is more senior than myself **[PS, CP – you balance your needs, and devise a feasible solution]**. Hence assessment and treatment can be initiated without me if necessary – even if there is an acute situation the GP can call an ambulance.

It ranks above Tasks C, D and E because there is potentially a higher risk to patient safety than with the other tasks. The patient may be acutely unwell, and there may be a drug on the discharge summary that has caused it, or may be used to treat it **[PS – you have thought around the issue, considering why it may be important]** – e.g. there may be details of a drug allergy and anaphylaxis reactions, which may help provide immediate life-saving treatment. There are also implications for relations with my colleagues **[PI]** – the GP is a key member of the team, and it is vital to help him or her provide optimal patient care. Moreover, I would be conscious **[CP]** of a senior colleague waiting for me on the phone. If there has been a serious problem as a result of a defect with the discharge summary, I would apologise to the GP **[CS, PI]**, and undertake a significant event analysis to learn from the event and prevent it recurring in future, even perhaps as part of an audit **[PS – again, you have thought around the issues and considered clinical governance]**.

More immediately I would consider delegating this task to do it quickly without stopping me from my vital ward tasks. **[CP, PS]** I could politely **[PI, CS]** ask my FY1 to do it if they were able to, explaining **[CS]** that I was very busy with ward jobs, and reassuring him that they could contact me if there were any problems **[PI]**. I could delegate to the ward-clerk, asking them to find out exactly what the GP required – if it was something simple like the discharge summary not being printed properly, the ward clerk could simply fax/email it, or read it out to the GP **[PS]**. I would thank **[CS, PI]** whoever I delegated the task to, and follow it up later to make sure it had been done **[PI]**.

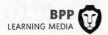

(3) TASK D

This task would initially worry me [PI – **you have recognised your own needs**] as there is a possibility that something untoward has happened to my partner, such as an accident. On the other hand, it may be something less sinister – e.g. they may want to let me know that they will be working late [PS – **dealing with uncertainty**]. I would rank this above Tasks C and E because the uncertainty would distract me from my work and cause me distress. My performance may be impaired and I may make serious mistakes relating to patient care, which may potentially cause harm [PI]. It also ranks highly because it can be done very quickly. I could make a very quick brief phone call, which may help reassure me that it is nothing serious [PS – **a workable, feasible solution**]. If it is serious but not urgent I could reassure [CS] my partner that I will see them as soon as possible after work. I could also delegate this to the ward-clerk, explaining the situation to them and politely [CS] ask them to call my partner to establish more facts [CP, PI]. If there is a serious and urgent issue, I would arrange ward cover with a colleague [PI], thanking them for their help [CS], then leave to see my partner.

Task D ranks below A and B because there is no immediate risk to anyone's life or safety at this point in time.

(4) TASK C

Task C ranks below A, B and D because there is no immediate risk to patient safety, as although the patient in question may be severely unwell they are stable.

It ranks above Task E because the consideration of relatives' views in relevant situations is good practice, as they may be aware of any advanced directives and the patient's views regarding end of life decisions [PS, PI – **you are trying to devise a feasible solution and are showing respect for others**]. This is essential to enable sound ethical judgements while respecting

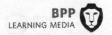

autonomy. Moreover, I could initially deal with the task [PS] by seeing the son and daughter and asking them to take a seat in a private comfortable place such as the patient's room. I would apologise for the delay [CS, PI], offering a cup of tea, while reassuring [CS] them that I will return as soon as possible. I could initially delegate this task, and consider asking [CS] a senior nurse or ward-sister who knows the patient well to start talking to the relatives [PS].

I do not know how terminal the patient's situation is, and whether or not they are competent to make decisions about their care [PS]. The patient may not want to discuss his illness with his children, [PS – **you are dealing with the uncertainty of the scenario**] in which case I would explain this to them while providing as much support and empathy [PI] as possible without compromising confidentiality until I am able to establish all of the facts.

(5) TASK E

I have ranked this task last because there is no immediate risk to patient safety. I appreciate that I have not been given details of the severity and nature of the patient affected, and importance of their medications. Obviously, intravenous antibiotics for an acutely sceptic elderly man would be a more pressing issue than aqueous cream for a stable person with mild eczema [PS]. However, from my experience, patients can usually be administered drugs as long as they are prescribed. I would check if the hospital policy permits this. Nevertheless, the task is very important because nurses may hesitate to administer drugs if they cannot document it, and this may delay the administration of vital medication [PI – **respect and consideration for your colleagues**], which would adversely affect patient care. It could also affect the performance of the nurses who are an instrumental part of the MDT, as they would be concerned about medicolegal implications of not documenting the drugs administered.

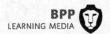

I would consider delegating this task to my FY1 or the ward pharmacist, explaining that I was very busy with other tasks, and then thanking **[CS]** them for their help **[PS, PI]**. I could also prioritise the drug charts, and immediately rewrite those with crucial medications, or those for severely unwell patients **[PS]**. Later, I could return to complete the remainder after more acute issues have been dealt with. In future I could suggest **[CS]** to my Consultant to initiate a policy that all junior doctors rewrite any drug charts nearing completion before the weekend **[PS]**, considering the heavy workload of the out of hours team.

Reflection: What have you learnt from this exercise?

I have learnt that all the tasks directly or indirectly affect the patient, and that I instinctively give most importance to patient care. I have also learnt the importance of recognising my own limitations and of asking for help when necessary. This is not only for my own individual needs, but also because factors affecting me would also affect my team and my patients. Another interesting point that emerged was that difficult tasks can only be prioritised well if a plan of action is devised, and if the multidisciplinary team is utilised effectively. The importance of following up tasks delegated to team members was also emphasised, as one can easily forget to ensure that tasks are completed when under pressure.

These answers to the tasks in Scenario A do not go through every single point discussed, as you will not have the time or space to elaborate on all of your thoughts. The key is to identify key topics and formulate a well-rounded answer that considers the problem, the NPS criteria, and the GMC's *Good Medical Practice* guidelines. The way you do this must demonstrate clear, logical and systematic thinking. This answer, together with the other practice scenarios contained in this book, aim to help you devise a framework and structure to enable you to cover the main points in your answer within the time available. You may have approached answering this scenario in a different way which could score just as well. The key is to justify your answers and take into account the GMC *Good Medical Practice* guidelines and the NPS criteria.

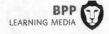

When reading through the answers to Scenario 1, consider the expressions used. A variety of words and phrases have been deliberately used to score highly on the 'Persuasive varied expression' sub-criterion. Rather than repeat the word 'immediate', 'at this moment in time' is used. You could also say 'in addition' or 'moreover' or 'as well as' to describe the same thing. 'Untoward' and 'sinister' are similar examples.

The way communication with colleagues and the patients has been demonstrated shows a considerate, sensitive and empathetic approach. In Task E the colleagues have been thanked for their assistance. In Task C when dealing with the patient's son and daughter, they were asked to sit down, and were apologised to for the delay in seeing them. Together with this the ward clerk was spoken to politely and the student nurse reassured. These are all buzzwords which will provide an impression that you actively ensure that you come across as sensitive to your colleagues and patients.

Practice scenarios

Now that you have worked through Scenario 1 there are a further nine scenarios for you to practise under timed conditions. Detailed discussions and answers are provided for Scenarios 2–5 and a summary overview is provided for Scenarios 6–10.

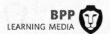

Practice Scenario 2

You are the Surgical SHO on-call in a busy District General Hospital on a Saturday. Your Registrar is in theatre, while your FY1 is on his way to a ward at the other end of the hospital to prescribe fluids for a pre-op patient. You step on to a ward and are immediately faced with a list of tasks.

Write the tasks in the order that you intend to rank them from 1 to 5, where 1 is the first task you would do, and 5 is the last. Write the letter of the task in the box provided. Justify your ranking and discuss any relevant issues relating to how you reached your decision. Write your answers within the box provided only.

At the start of the exercise you will be given five minutes to read the question, during which you will not be allowed to write. Following this you will have 20 minutes to complete your answers in the boxes provided.

(A) The A&E sister bleeps to inform you that a patient referred to you by a GP has arrived. He has severe abdominal pain and the nurse wants you to see him immediately.

(B) A staff nurse from an orthopaedic ward would like a patient recovering from a hip replacement to be reviewed. He has been confused for the last six hours since this morning.

(C) Your daughter's babysitter has left a message saying that she is unwell, and has asked you to ring back immediately.

(D) A nurse would like you to see a patient who wants to self discharge.

(E) The hospital security guard has rung the ward demanding that you move your car, as it is parked illegally and will be clamped if not moved immediately.

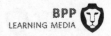

1. TASK
2. TASK
3. TASK
4. TASK
5. TASK
Reflection: What did you find easiest about this exercise?

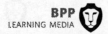

Suggested Approach to Scenario 2

Categorise the tasks:

- Definite immediate danger to life (I)
- Possible danger to life (P)
- Unlikely danger to life (U)

Task A

The A&E sister bleeps to inform you that a patient referred to you by a GP has arrived. He has severe abdominal pain and the nurse wants you to see him immediately.

There is a strong possibility that a patient referred to the surgical team with an acute abdominal pain may have a life threatening condition such as bowel obstruction or a ruptured perforated ulcer. However, remember that this patient is in an A&E department, and is probably surrounded by several A&E doctors and nurses who have the best resources in the hospital to deal with a medical or surgical emergency. Many of the doctors will be more experienced than you and better trained to deal with emergencies, so there may not necessarily be much that you can do. You could choose to categorise this task as I, as there is a significant possibility of an immediate risk to life. In view of the fact that the patient is in A&E, you could also categorise it as P.

Task B

A staff nurse from an orthopaedic ward would like a patient recovering from a hip replacement to be reviewed. He has been confused for the last six hours since this morning.

There could be a number of reasons for the confusion, and the implications of limited information are clearly evident in this case. There are many serious pathologies that could result in confusion, ranging from sepsis to a stroke. Without this information one has to consider the worst-case scenario, which is that the confusion may be caused by a life-threatening condition which needs urgent treatment so this could be categorised as I.

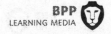

Task C

Your daughter's babysitter has left a message saying that she is unwell, and has asked you to ring back immediately.

This is the 'personal' task, so again you need to decide how you would react. Knowing that your daughter is with a babysitter, you may be able to put this task aside and call after your other tasks have been completed, which would designate this task a U. However, you may find yourself very distressed to the extent that your performance and subsequent patient care become affected, in which case you could categorise it as P. It depends on how you would react as an individual.

Task D

A nurse would like you to see a patient who wants to self discharge.

You do not know why this patient wishes to self-discharge. They may have a medical or psychiatric problem that render them incompetent, in which case they may need to be sectioned and restrained. You cannot deduce what their underlying problem is until they are reviewed. However, ensure you read the scenario carefully – it states that the patient wants to discharge. This implies that they are not trying to leave forcibly, therefore this task could be categorised as P.

Task E

The hospital security guard has rung the ward demanding that you move your car, as it is parked illegally and will be clamped if not moved immediately.

This task has important implications for teamwork and your relations with your colleagues. There is a small possibility that your car is blocking the ambulance pathway, or something else which has an impact on patient safety. This will cause huge inconvenience to the ambulance crews, or whoever you are blocking. Nevertheless it is almost always possible to work around a car causing a blockage, and this task is not directly related to patient safety. Hence, this task could be categorised as a U.

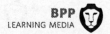

Categories and ranking:

Task A	P	Rank 2nd or 3rd
Task B	I	Rank 1st
Task C	P/U	Rank 4th
Task D	P	Rank 2nd or 3rd
Task E	U	Rank 5th

Task B

A staff nurse from an orthopaedic ward would like a patient recovering from a hip replacement to be reviewed. He has been confused for the last six hours since this morning.

Limited information – best and worst case scenarios
- The patient may be unstable from a stroke, pulmonary embolism, or severe sepsis.
- The nurse may be new to the ward, and unaware that the patient has chronic dementia.

Who does it affect?
(a) Patient: If he or she has a serious acute underlying condition.
(b) Team:
   - The staff-nurse who called you
   - Your seniors, such as the surgical or even medical or ITU Registrar
   - Ward nurses
(c) Yourself: This may be a time consuming, stressful task.
(d) Other issues:
   Education: If the patient is not confused, the nurse may have a learning need on how to identify and manage acute confusion.
   Hospital policy: If the nurse did not know that the patient has chronic confusion or dementia, she may have not received a proper handover. A clear and comprehensive handover system needs to be incorporated into the hospital policy.

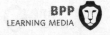

Using the MDT

If you review the patient immediately and find that the confusion is acute and secondary to a serious condition you could institute treatment immediately. If you feel you need to confirm that your management plan is appropriate with a senior, you could leave a message with the theatre nurse asking your surgical Registrar to contact you after they have finished. If it is more urgent, you could go there yourself and see if they would be happy to talk to you while operating. If the problem is not surgical, you may want to talk to the medical or ITU Registrar on-call, explaining that your own Registrar is in theatre. In the interim it would be prudent to consult the staff nurse or ward sister when devising your management plan.

If you were busy with something even more important, you could delegate to your FY1 to make an initial assessment. Alternatively, you could ask the nurse to collate important information which you could use to devise your management plan, such as the observations, while reassuring them that you will come as soon as possible.

On the other hand, the patient may be chronically confused with dementia. In this case you need to reassure the nurse who called you, and later explore whether identifying confusion is one of their learning needs, and work with them constructively to address this. If the nurse did make a mistake, they may be deterred from calling requesting your assistance in the future, so you need to reassure them that you are happy to be contacted later if there are any concerns.

Follow-up

If the confusion is acute, you should return later and review the patient to ensure that they are stable and improving. You may also need to handover the patient to the night team, for monitoring or follow-up. If the medical or ITU team are involved, clarify whether or not they intend to follow up the patient. You may decide to audit handover problems and take this up as a policy issue with the clinical governance administrators.

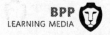

Recognising limitations

- Time and workload: You may have to enlist the help of the nursing staff, or delegate to the FY1.
- Clinical acumen: You may need someone who is more senior and experienced to assess and manage the patient.

Comparing the tasks

The first and last ranked tasks are usually easy to justify. This task ranks above all others because there is potentially an immediate life threatening problem that needs addressing by a doctor.

Task D

Limited information – best and worst case scenarios

A nurse would like you to see a patient who wants to self discharge.

- A stable patient: they may just be waiting for medications or a social care package that can be organised after discharge.
- An unstable patient: they may have a serious condition for which hospital based life-saving treatment is essential, such as intravenous antibiotics, fluids or oxygen.
- An incompetent patient, for example, if they have a psychiatric disorder.

Who does it affect?

(a) Patient: They may put their own life at risk if vital hospital treatment is denied, or even other individuals if they are aggressive and incompetent. Their autonomy and legal rights will be violated if they are competent and forced to stay against their wishes. If there is a vocal argument on the wards the other patients will be affected.

(b) Team:
- The nurse who called you.
- Anyone involved in the patients discharge – e.g. pharmacists, ward nurses etc.

(c) Yourself: This may be a time-consuming and stressful task.

(d) Other issues:
- Hospital and NHS reputation: if there is a loud argument between the patient and the nurse.
- Ethics: as discussed above.

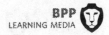

Using the MDT

The nurse has just bleeped you. The most prudent course of action would be to obtain as many details regarding the patient as you can. Why was the patient admitted? Why do they want to leave? How are they clinically? A useful starting point generally is the observations chart. Can their treatment only be administered in hospital? When are they due to be discharged? If the nurse is a ward-sister, or a senior ward based nurse who knows the patient well, they may be able to clarify that the patient is fully competent, is only waiting for his medications, and needs to see his spouse who has been involved in a car accident. In such a case you could consider discharging the patient, and discuss the options available with the nurse to ensure a safe and well organised discharge. You may negotiate a solution with the patient whereby they see their GP soon after discharge. They may be able to return to the ward later to collect their medications. If you think laterally and utilise all the resources and MDT members at your disposal, you may not even need to go to the ward at all.

The patient may be angry or irate because of something that has happened on the ward, or perhaps they have had an altercation with a nurse or another member of the MDT. You would need to be tactful in your approach, and the key is empathy and sensitivity. Regardless of what the patient is saying it always helps to listen initially without saying anything for the first few minutes. You should also adopt a similar approach with the nurse. Consider the effect of this in the nurse, who may be feeling demoralised or angry. This will also have a knock-on effect on the patient care provided by the nurse. Showing empathy and sensitivity, while offering to come and talk to the nurse may help. Above all be objective, and help both – never take sides in such a situation, as it will only make things worse!

The patient may have been admitted due to a serious life-threatening illness. If they are adamant on leaving, you may have to make a clinical assessment and talk to the patient about the risks associated with discharge. As discussed above, the situation may become more complex if they are incompetent. You will probably have to call your seniors, such as your Registrar or even your Consultant for their advice. The psychiatry team may also need to get involved. The

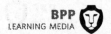

patient may even become violent, so you may need to assistance from the security personnel.

Follow-up

This is relevant only if you agree to see the patient or the ward nurse later on.

Recognising limitations

- Clinical acumen: To assess whether the patient can be safely discharged.
- Mental Health Act: Sectioning requires doctors with a specific amount of experience and qualifications.

Comparing the tasks

This task ranks above Tasks A, C and E because the patient may be severely unwell. Their life may be at risk without hospital treatment, or they may have a serious underlying pathology causing confusion or a psychiatric disturbance. The patient in Task A is in a place where there are staff and facilities to make an assessment and start treatment. There appears to be no obvious life-threatening event in tasks C or E. It ranks below Task B because one can reasonably infer that the patient in this task is clinically stable enough to talk to the nurse and decide to self-discharge.

Task A

The A&E sister bleeps to inform you that a patient referred to you by a GP has arrived. He has severe abdominal pain and the nurse wants you to see him immediately.

Limited information – best and worst case scenarios

- Acute life-threatening condition: such as acute bowel obstruction, a perforated duodenal ulcer, acute cholecystitis and so on.
- Non-life threatening cause: such as severe chronic constipation.

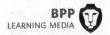

The advantage here is that the patient is in A&E and under the jurisdiction of the team there, who could assess and stabilise him if required.

Who does it affect?

(a) Patient: As above.
(b) Team:
- A&E sister
- A&E doctors.
(c) Yourself: Again, this is may be a stressful task that requires significant input.
(d) Other issues:
A&E Management: It is imperative to appreciate the effects of the patients waiting in A&E departments, which are often busy and overstretched. The four-hour target is also important, as the patient may breach it, resulting in major financial implications for the Trust.

Using the MDT

Start by liaising with the A&E sister who has contacted you, and find out how they would like you to help. A&E has plenty of doctors with specialist skills and facilities in dealing with acutely unwell patients, and you could utilise these to good effect. The surgical Registrar may be needed if the patient urgently needs an operation.

Even if you see the patient, you could delegate several tasks, such as phlebotomy, to the A&E staff including the nurses. If the patient is stable, your FY1 may be able to clerk them.

Follow-up

If the patient remains in A&E, you will need to follow them up and carry out a surgical review. If you ask your FY1 to review them, you need to contact him to see how they are progressing.

Recognising limitations

- Time and workload: manage by delegation as above.
- Clinical limitations: liaise with A&E seniors or your Registrar.

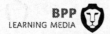

Comparing the tasks

This task ranks above Tasks C and E because there are direct implications for patient safety, and it can also be dealt with very quickly if you work with your colleagues both in the surgical team and in A&E. It ranks below Tasks B and D because the patient is in A&E which is well equipped by staff and facilities to cope with emergencies.

Task C

Your daughter's babysitter has left a message saying that she is unwell, and has asked you to ring back immediately.

Limited information – best and worst case scenarios

This depends on you. What comes to your mind?

- Your daughter's life may be in danger and she may need hospitalisation.
- She may have something far less serious such as chicken pox.

Who does it affect?

(a) Patient: If your concentration is hindered and you make mistakes, patient safety may be compromised.

(b) Team: As with the patient, the team function will also be hindered.

(c) Yourself: As with all the personal tasks, the most significant effect of this scenario will be on yourself. You have emotional needs, and you may need help in dealing with these. You may want to go to attend to your daughter immediately, or at least ring the babysitter and find out what is going on. On the other hand you may be of the view that the babysitter would have taken the child to hospital if it was necessary.

(d) Other issues:
    Medical staffing: to organise cover if you have to leave.

Using the MDT

If you are in the middle of a task, you could ask the administrative staff, such as the ward-clerk, to ring the babysitter and take a message after explaining your situation to them.

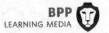

If you are required to attend your daughter, you will have to find someone to cover your absence by liaising with your seniors, in particular the surgical Registrar. The hospital managers would also have to be consulted.

Follow-up

If you ask someone to ring the babysitter, then you should obviously get back to them and find out the reason for the call. Likewise, if you tell your babysitter that you will call her back, it is imperative that you do so.

Recognising limitations

- Emotional limitations: Even the most thick-skinned of people become anxious when they are concerned about their young children. It is vital to recognise these implications on patient care.

Comparing the tasks

This task ranks above Task E because it has significant emotional effects, as well as knock-on effects for patient safety. It can also be potentially dealt with very quickly. It ranks below the other tasks because there is no immediate danger to anyone's life.

Task E

The hospital security guard has rung the ward demanding that you move your car, as it is parked illegally and will be clamped if not moved immediately.

Limited information - best and worst case scenarios

- You are blocking the A&E pathway. Even then, it is certainly not impossible to bring patients into A&E from the ambulance, although the inconvenience caused to your colleagues will be considerable.
- Your car is parked in a space reserved for someone else.

Who does it affect?

(a) Patient: This is unlikely to have any major effects on patients, even if you are blocking the ambulance pathway, as they

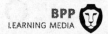

will probably find another way to bring patients in from the ambulance.

(b) Team:
- The security attendant who called you.
- Other team members, such as the ambulance drivers.

(c) Yourself: There is probably a fine for clamping, and this may distract you from your work.

(d) Other issues:
Hospital policy: Contravening any hospital rules and regulations is not advisable, although we all make mistakes.

Using the MDT

If you are in the middle of something vital, such as a procedure, you could ask the ward clerk to ring security and notify them that you will move your car as soon as possible. If they are very busy you could ring them yourself. This can be done quickly within a couple of minutes.

Follow-up

Unless you move your car immediately, all the other options require you to move your car later on at some point.

Recognising limitations

There is no real scope to recognise limitations in this task.

Comparing the tasks

This ranks last because it does not put anyone's life at risk, and has minimal effect on the patient, yourself and your ward team. This is not to undermine the importance of the problem it causes for the security attendant, who is a vital part of the team.

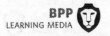

Suggested Answer for Scenario 2

(1) TASK B

This ranks highest because it presents the most immediate risk to patient safety if the confusion is acute and secondary to a life-threatening illness. To determine this, I will have to review the patient and ask the nurse to collate vital information such as observations while I was on my way. If I felt that I lacked the expertise needed to manage the patient alone, I would ask a senior, such as a Registrar, for their help. This may be from the medical, surgical or ITU specialties, depending on which domain the illness fell under. If after assessing the patient, I felt that his condition was not as serious, I could delegate it to my FY1 explaining my ward jobs, and asking him to feed back to me once he was done. I would also thank the nurse who called me, and would consult her when devising a management strategy as she may be implementing it. If the patient was chronically confused e.g. due to dementia, I would feed this back to the nurse, and explore why she was concerned or did not receive a comprehensive handover in a constructive manner, while reassuring her that she could contact me if she had any concerns about anyone later on.

(2) TASK D

This task ranks above A, C and E because the patient may be severely unwell and confused, causing him to want to self-discharge. I would assess them, and explore the reasons for him wanting to self-discharge, and try to negotiate a compromise to convince the patient to stay until his treatment is complete. However, if they are competent and adamant to leave despite my explanation of the risks, I would respect his autonomy and allow him to go, asking him to sign a self-discharge form in accordance with the hospital policy. I would also offer to call my senior as this may reassure him. If he is stable and does not require hospital treatment, I may just talk to him over the phone, and discharge him and arrange follow-up. If there was a senior nurse on the ward who could confirm all this, I could ask her to do this as she may know the patient better than me, while explaining why it would be difficult for me to see the patient.

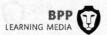

The patient may be incompetent, and confused due to an organic or psychiatric disorder. I will try to calmly and reassuringly convince the patient to stay- if he did not, I may consider sectioning him under the Mental Health Act, and ask my seniors (including a psychiatry Registrar), to review the patient.

(3) TASK A

This task ranks below the Tasks B and D because the patient is in A&E which is the best place for acutely unwell patients, with respect to the specialist doctors and nurses, and also the facilities. It ranks above Tasks C and E because there is a possibility of a direct imminent risk to patient safety. First, I would find out why the nurse is contacting me. She may be merely informing me that the patient referred to the surgical team has arrived, and that he is stable and does not need an urgent review. I would thank her for the call, and reassure her that I will be there as soon as possible. If the patient is unwell and requires surgical intervention, he requires an urgent review, although it is likely that an A&E senior, such as a Registrar would have seen him as the patient falls under the jurisdiction of A&E while he is there. Even if surgery is required, they will probably contact the surgical Registrar directly, as most A&E Registrars are more experienced and senior than myself. If the A&E staff are busy and need me to review the patient, I could do this efficiently by delegating tasks such as phlebotomy to the A&E nurses, and asking them politely to collate vital information before I arrive. A quick initial assessment may be enough to conclude that the patient is relatively stable, in which case I may ask my FY1 to do a full clerking and report back to me.

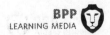

(4) TASK C

I have ranked this task above Task E because the message would make me worry, and the emotional impact may compromise the patient care I provide. I have ranked it below the others because the risk to patient safety is not as acute. Ideally, I would like to ring back immediately and find out exactly what the problem is. If the problem is not urgent, this call could take only a couple of minutes relieving any worry in the process. I would explain to the babysitter that I am on-call, and offer to ring her back as soon as my shift finishes. Alternatively, I could text or ring my spouse, or a close friend asking him or her to contact the babysitter.

If something serious has happened to my daughter I would be too distressed to continue working, and would have to leave and go to her. I would explain this to my seniors and liaise with the management team to organise cover. I would also apologise to my colleagues, and provide a comprehensive handover, reassuring them that they could ring me on my mobile if they require information about any patient I had seen earlier.

(5) TASK E

This ranks below the other tasks because it involves no risk to anyone's life, and has the least effect on the patients and my team. However I appreciate that it is a professional requirement to adhere to hospital rules and regulations, and that not doing so may hinder the work of the security attendants. I would try to resolve it by ideally moving my car as soon as possible, and apologising to the attendant. However if I was in the middle of a vital job, I would politely ask the ward clerk if she could inform security that I would be there as soon as I could. I also appreciate that I may be blocking an important point of access, such as the ambulance pathway which would hinder the work of the ambulance staff. In this case I would also apologise to them.

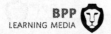

Reflection: What did you find easiest about this exercise?

The easiest part of this exercise was deciding which task should be ranked last. Some of the tasks have serious immediate effects on patient safety, while others affect my team or myself in important ways. However the effects of task E on my patients, my team and myself are minimal and non-immediate. Nevertheless, I recognise its importance as I have discussed in the box above, and it is ranked last only in relative terms. Generally, I prioritise the tasks by identifying any factors that put anyone's life at immediate risk (patients or staff). This should obviously be dealt with first. I then stratify the tasks by evaluating the effects on my patients, my team and myself. Using such a method makes it easy to discriminate between tasks which need to be dealt with immediately from others which are less urgent.

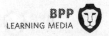

Practice Scenario 3

You are the doctor-on-triage for your GP practice as a GPST1. It is an exceptionally busy Friday. Decide how you will prioritise these tasks.

Write the tasks in the order that you intend to rank them from 1 to 5, where 1 is the first task you would do, and 5 is the last. Write the letter of the task in the box provided. Justify your ranking and discuss any relevant issues relating to how you reached your decision. Write your answers within the box provided only.

At the start of the exercise you will be given five minutes to read the question, during which you will not be allowed to write. Following this you will have 20 minutes to complete your answers in the boxes provided.

(A) The wife of a 74-year-old patient calls you angrily demanding a home visit for her husband as he has had a fall.

(B) The FY1 telephones you from another room for help because his patient is becoming loud and aggressive.

(C) The practice pharmacist is calling you as it is time for the monthly audit meeting.

(D) The receptionists call you because a patient is getting 'really short of breath' in the waiting room.

(E) Your spouse has left a message on your answer-phone asking you to ring back. She sounds very upset.

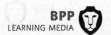

1.   TASK
2.   TASK
3.   TASK
4.   TASK
5.   TASK
Reflection: What two things would you do differently next time?

Suggested Approach to Scenario 3

Categorise the tasks:

* Definite immediate danger to life (I)
* Possible danger to life (P)
* Unlikely danger to life (U)

Task A

The wife of a 74-year-old patient calls you angrily demanding a home visit for her husband as he has had a fall.

We have no details about the reason for the home visit. The wife has not said that he is unconscious or has any immediately life-threatening condition. Nevertheless, he may have sustained a fracture, or have a serious underlying condition causing the fall. Hence, this task could be categorised as a P.

Task B

The FY1 telephones you from another room for help because his patient is becoming loud and aggressive.

Most practices have a panic button, and you could be reassured that the FY1 has not used this because he does not feel in danger. Alternatively, he may be unaware of its existence. One may also argue that if he is able to pick up the phone and dial your number the patient is probably not violent at the moment, although they may become violent soon if no action is taken. There is a potential risk to the FY1's well being, although probably not immediately, therefore this task can be categorised as a P.

Task C

The practice pharmacist is calling you as it is time for the monthly audit meeting.

There is no risk to anyone's life imminently, so this task can be categorised as a U.

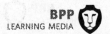

Task D

The receptionists call you because a patient is getting 'really short of breath' in the waiting room.

Any problems with the airway are urgent, as defined by the ALS guidelines and the ABC guidelines. The receptionists are not trained to assess or manage this, so this task can be categorised as an I.

Task E

Your spouse has left a message on your answer-phone asking you to ring back. She sounds very upset.

As always, the personal task may affect your care of patients indirectly if you are emotionally distressed. There is no risk to patients other than your frame of mind therefore this task can be categorised as a P or U.

Categories and ranking:

Task A	P	Rank 2nd or 3rd
Task B	P	Rank 2nd or 3rd
Task C	U	Rank 5th
Task D	I	Rank 1st
Task E	P/U	Rank 4th

Task D

The receptionists call you because a patient is getting 'really short of breath' in the waiting room.

Limited information – best and worst case scenarios

- The patient may be experiencing acute airway obstruction, such as an anaphylactic shock.
- The patient may be obese and generally unfit albeit not acutely unwell and be panting due to rushing to the surgery to avoid being late.

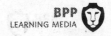

Who does it affect?

(a) Patient: In the worst case scenario, the patient may die very quickly without intervention.

(b) Team:
   •   The receptionist who called you.

(c) Yourself: Possibly a time-consuming task.

(d) Other issues: None.

Using the MDT

You must review this patient immediately – this cannot be delegated. If the patient is in extremis, you will probably want to ask other GPs to help you initiate management. If he is close to cardiac arrest, you may shout to call someone with specialist resuscitation skills, such as the juniors who have recently completed hospital placements and life-support courses or nurses trained in resuscitation. The receptionist could call an ambulance.

Follow-up

If you find that the patient is not very short of breath, you could see him briefly and come back to him to make sure he is being seen to.

Recognising limitations

•   Clinical acumen: Your seniors will have more experience of dealing with emergencies in primary care, and your colleagues with resuscitation training may be more up to date with airway management techniques.

•   Time and workload: You are still the triage doctor. If other GPs who are less busy can manage the patient, you could leave and continue your triage work.

Comparing the tasks

This is potentially a case of airway obstruction and therefore poses the greatest threat to patient safety.

Task B

The FY1 telephones you from another room for help because his patient is becoming loud and aggressive.

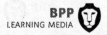

Limited information – best and worst case scenarios

- The patient may be irate and annoyed, but not angry or aggressive at all.
- The patient may have an underlying psychiatric disorder, and may be on the verge of becoming seriously violent due to an exacerbation of their condition.

Who does it affect?

(a) Patient: If they have an underlying disorder which is causing their aggression, they may put themselves and others at risk.

(b) Team:
- The FY1 doctor calling you.

(c) Yourself: Again, this is another potentially stressful task that requires significant input.

(d) Other issues:

Practice policy: All practices have a policy for dealing with potentially violent patients – this often involves a panic alarm. If the FY1 is not aware of this, there may be a problem with the induction programme for new doctors. If there is no such policy, this needs to be addressed and one needs to be devised as soon as possible.

Significant Event Analysis: An FY1 having to call someone to help deal with a potentially violent patient is unacceptable.

Using the MDT

If the patient is potentially violent, you may need support from your colleagues to physically restrain the patient if required. In this case, you will probably need the police involved as well, who the receptionists can call.

Follow-up

If the patient is mildly aggressive, you could calm them down, then go back to the FY1 and make sure there are no further problems.

Recognising limitations

- Time and workload: manage by delegation.

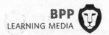

- Physical limitations: seriously angry and violent patients usually need more than one person to restrain them. You could utilise anyone suitable for this purpose.

Comparing the tasks

This task ranks above Tasks C and E because someone's well-being is potentially in danger. It ranks above Task A because it can be dealt with more quickly as you are in the practice. It ranks below D because the risk to life is less immediate.

Task A

The wife of a 74-year-old patient calls you angrily demanding a home visit for her husband as he has had a fall.

Limited information – best and worst case scenarios

- The patient may be lying on the floor with a fractured hip with severe internal bleeding.
- He may have had the fall because of a severe systemic illness, such as dehydration secondary to sepsis, or poor co-ordination because of a stroke.
- It may just be a mechanical fall, and he may have got back up and started walking immediately.

Who does it affect?

(a) Patient: This depends on which of the three options above applies in this case.
(b) Team:
    - Currently no members of the team are affected.
(c) Yourself: Time consuming, logistically difficult task.
(d) Other issues: None.

Using the MDT

There may already be a doctor conducting a home visit near the patient's home, and they may be able to add this patient to their list. If an acute condition has caused the fall or results from the fall, you may need to call an ambulance or ask the patient to go to hospital. You could refer him directly to the relevant team, such as orthopaedics (e.g. if he has a fracture) or medicine (if he

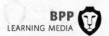

has severe dehydration or a stroke causing the fall). If the patient sounds reasonably well, it may be more appropriate to ask a junior doctor (such as a FY1) or a district nurse to review him. If he is mobile and ambulant you could add him on to a GP's list in the afternoon surgery.

Follow-up

If you ask a district nurse or junior doctor to visit him, you should ask them to report back to you.

Recognising limitations

- Time and workload: As triage doctor you should be able to appropriately delegate the assessment of this patient, although it will take time to do this properly.
- Staffing: There is limited number of doctors and nurses, and the necessity for a home visit should be considered carefully.

Comparing the tasks

This task ranks above Task A and C because it is directly related to patient safety. It ranks below the others because it is unlikely that the patient's life is in immediate danger.

Task E

Your spouse has left a message on your answer-phone asking you to ring back. She sounds very upset.

Limited information – best and worst case scenarios

- A deeply distressing event has occurred affecting your spouse, such as the bereavement of a close relative.
- She may not be upset at all, and you may have misinterpreted her tone of voice.

Who does it affect?

(a) Patient: As with all personal tasks, your emotional distress will reflect on your clinical management, and patient safety may be at risk especially as you are the triage doctor determining which patients are acutely unwell.

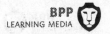

(b) Team:
   - Currently no one from the team is being affected.
(c) Yourself: You will be emotionally strained as a result of the uncertainty regarding your spouse, and the nature of her message. This will impair your concentration and your decision making abilities, and you may miss diagnoses and not prescribe safely. Patient safety may be compromised.
(d) Other issues: None.

Using the MDT

The receptionist could call your spouse and take a message on your behalf. If you do ring back and circumstances dictate that you have to leave, you should talk to your trainer or other senior GPs as well as the practice manager and help them arrange cover, with a comprehensive handover of what you have done so far.

Follow-up

If you leave, you could ring later to find out how the practice coped without you, and whether there is anything that requires clarifying. If you decide to ring your spouse later on, remember to actually do this.

Recognising limitations

- Emotional limitations: Depending on your personal circumstances not establishing whether there is a serious problem may impact on your frame of mind and affect the quality of your work.

Comparing the tasks

This task ranks below Tasks D, B and A because there is no immediate risk to anyone's life. It ranks above Task C because patient care may be affected indirectly, and also because it could be dealt with very quickly if it emerges that your spouse has no immediate serious issue.

Task C

The practice pharmacist is calling you as it is time for the monthly audit meeting.

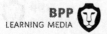

Limited information – best and worst case scenarios

- There may be serious issues relating to patient safety that have been identified in an audit.
- There may be no significant recommendations from any of the audits to date.

Who does it affect?

(a) Patient: In the longer term, the audit will help improve standards of patient care.

(b) Team:
   - The Practice Manager: who organises the meetings and has probably arranged for this time as per availability of the team members, including you.
   - The receptionists: who may be taking calls while the doctors are in the meeting.

(c) Yourself: You will benefit from the recommendations of the audit as this will impact positively on your patient care. However, being the triage doctor on a busy day like this, attending the meeting may deprive you of valuable time which you need to deal with more urgent issues.

(d) Other issues:
   Clinical governance: Audits are tools to improve standards of clinical care. This applies individually, collectively and systemically (with respect to the infrastructure and management of the practice).

Using the MDT

The practice pharmacist could provide you with the minutes of the meeting or individually discuss the findings and recommendations of the audit with you. You could ask the Practice Manager for copies of any handouts. Another GP could replace you as triage doctor while you attend part of the meeting. The receptionist could take calls and ask non-urgent callers to ring back later on.

Follow-up

If you attend the meeting, you will have to ensure that any missed calls are returned. If you do not attend, you should find out about the main points raised at the meeting to improve your own practice.

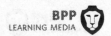

Recognising limitations
- Time and workload: as discussed, attending the meeting will deprive you of vital time and increase your workload.

Comparing the tasks

This task ranks last because there will be no immediate effects on patient care, and it is quite time consuming. Nevertheless, clinical governance and constantly striving to improve practice and maintain high standards of care is a requirement of professional development.

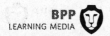

Suggested Answer for Scenario 3

(1) TASK D

I need to assess this patient as there may be a direct and immediate risk to his life which therefore means I would rank this task first. I will follow the A-B-C guidelines, and if I find that any of these are compromised, I will immediately request help from my colleagues. I will involve my seniors, and any doctors or nurses who have resuscitation training as they may be more adept than me at managing such an emergency. I would ask the receptionist to call an ambulance. Later, if my colleagues are happy to manage the patient without me, I may leave and continue my work as triage doctor, as there may well be other sick patients.

If the patient is not extremely unwell, e.g. if he has mild asthma, I would request a practice nurse or another doctor to see the patient, while explaining that I had many jobs to do, thanking them for their help. If the patient was fine, I would thank the receptionists for alerting me, and reassure them that they could notify me if they had any further concerns.

(2) TASK B

This task ranks below D because the potential risk to life is less immediate. If the patient was violent, the FY1 would have been unable to pick up the phone, dial my number and ring me. If it emerges that the patient is relatively calm I would try to diffuse the situation quickly, and reassure the FY1 that they could contact me again if they had any further concerns. Later I may ask a senior GP to make sure that the FY1 was not having any further problems, explaining that I was busy with my triage-doctor duties.

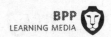

I have ranked this above the other tasks, because there is a possibility of threat to the FY1's well-being if the patient was becoming violent. If this was the case I would follow practice policy and press the panic-button (or equivalent), and ask for immediate assistance from my colleagues to restrain the patient. If necessary, I would also ask the receptionists to call the police. Later, I would constructively explore why the FY1 had to ring me. Either the practice policy is inadequate to deal with angry violent patients, or this was missing from the FY1's induction programme. I would raise this at the next Significant Event Analysis meeting.

(3) TASK A

This task ranks above E and C because there may be a direct risk to patient safety. My first priority would be to whether the patient was clinically stable. A few quick questions could determine this – e.g. is he walking around? Is he eating and talking? Is he in any pain? The patient may be unstable as a result of the fall (e.g. if he has fractured his hip), or as a result of the cause (e.g. dehydration secondary to sepsis). If this is the case, I could send an ambulance to the patient's house while advising the wife on how to manage him in the interim.

If the patient was stable (e.g. if he had a mechanical fall with no obvious major injury) I would explore the wife's reasons for demanding a home visit, and express empathy and sensitivity towards her perspective. If the patient was able to come to the surgery, I would book him into a colleague's afternoon surgery. If not, I could ask one of the district nurses or junior doctors to visit him if his condition was not very severe and reassure her that they could ring me for advice if needed. If the condition was more complex, I could ask one of the GPs to visit him, preferably one who was in the area anyway.

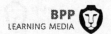

(4) TASK E

This task ranks above C, because there is an indirect risk to patient safety depending on how the situation affected me. I would be very concerned about my spouse if she sounded upset and had left an unusual message for me. This would hinder my decision making and concentration, and could hinder my patient care. I could deal with it quickly by ringing her immediately and allaying my uncertainty by finding out what the problem is. If it was non-urgent, I would reassure my partner and offer to ring back at the end of surgery. If it was a serious issue and I had to leave the surgery, I would explain the reasons to my Practice Manager and my trainer, and help them organise cover, thanking them for their co-operation. I could also request to the receptionist to call my spouse and take a message if I was busy.

(5) TASK C

This task ranks last because it does not immediately affect anyone's safety, and is time consuming. In view of the tasks, I may not attend the meeting today. Nevertheless, I recognise its importance in helping me improve my clinical standards and to identify any problems with current practice. I could ask the practice pharmacist if she could talk to me about the audits at a later date, or provide me with a copy of the handouts, after explaining and apologising for my absence. On the other hand I could negotiate with another doctor to take over triage from me while I was in the meeting, and perhaps attend half of it. I could also ask the reception staff to ask all non-urgent callers to call after the meeting and take any messages for me, while thanking them for their help.

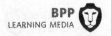

Reflection: What two things would you do differently next time?

First, I would try to maximise the educational dividends from my experience by identifying learning needs and ways to address these. There is immense educational benefit to be derived from a busy day like this with multiple difficult tasks to be completed in a limited duration of time. I would try to identify both clinical and non-clinical issues, and go through these with my trainer. During my next 'on-call' day I would compare my performance to today's and reflect on how I have improved.

Second, I would consider asking one of my senior colleagues for help with the 'duty-triage' work earlier on. I relish the responsibility placed on me as the 'triage-doctor' on-call, but it is also vital to recognise limitations and adapt to a situation in accordance with the circumstances. There is a possibility that the day is too busy for only one doctor on-call to deal with, especially considering that he or she is the most junior member of the team. Discussing this with a senior colleague would not only provide assistance for the jobs, but also help me develop new methods and strategies to cope with them.

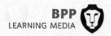

Practice Scenario 4

You are an FY2 in General Practice, and have your own surgery on a busy Friday evening approaching Christmas. You are near the end of your surgery, and suddenly seem to have many jobs to do.

Write the tasks in the order that you intend to rank them from 1 to 5, where 1 is the first task you would do, and 5 is the last. Write the letter of the task in the box provided. Justify your ranking and discuss any relevant issues relating to how you reached your decision. Write your answers within the box provided only.

At the start of the exercise you will be given five minutes to read the question, during which you will not be allowed to write. Following this you will have 20 minutes to complete your answers in the boxes provided.

(A) There is a Drug Representative waiting to speak to you about a new form of simvastatin available on the market.

(B) Your GP Trainer would like to go through your Personal Development Plan as part of your e-portfolio.

(C) The receptionist phones you because she is concerned about a patient in the waiting room who is vomiting profusely.

(D) The practice nurse would like you to see an asthmatic who she has put on a salbutamol nebulizer.

(E) A patient with disseminated bowel cancer phones you from home asking for a prescription of painkillers.

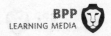

1.   TASK
2.   TASK
3.   TASK
4.   TASK
5.   TASK
Reflection: What limitations in your own skills did you identify from this?

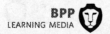

Suggested Approach to Scenario 4

Categorise the tasks:

- Definite immediate danger to life (I)
- Possible danger to life (P)
- Unlikely danger to life (U)

Task A

There is a Drug Representative waiting to speak to you about a new form of simvastatin available on the market.

There is obviously no danger to life so therefore this task can be categorised as a U.

Task B

Your GP Trainer would like to go through your Personal Development Plan as part of your e-portfolio.

There is no risk to life here either so therefore this task can be categorised as a U.

Task C

The receptionist phones you because she is concerned about a patient in the waiting room who is vomiting profusely.

Severe vomiting can be the cause or effect of a serious condition, such as severe bacterial gastroenteritis, so you could categorise this task as a P. However, they may even be vomiting blood, in which case it would be life threatening. So you argue that this task should be categorised as an I.

Task D

The practice nurse would like you to see an asthmatic woman who she has put on a salbutamol nebulizer.

This patient's asthma is severe enough to warrant a nebulizer. However, if they were unstable, the practice nurse would have probably drawn your attention to this, or would have asked another

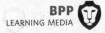

doctor to see the patient. As the patient is being attended to by a fellow medical professional and treatment has been initiated, the risk to their safety is probably not immediate and can therefore be categorised as a P.

Task E

A patient with disseminated bowel cancer phones you from home asking for a prescription of painkillers.

There is unlikely to be any new imminent risk to the patient's life as it sounds like they are receiving palliative care. Hence this could be ranked as a U.

Categories and ranking:

Task A	U	Rank 3rd, 4th or 5th
Task B	U	Rank 3rd, 4th or 5th
Task C	I	Rank 1st
Task D	P	Rank 2nd
Task E	U	Rank 3rd, 4th or 5th

Task C

The receptionist phones you because she is concerned about a patient in the waiting room who is vomiting profusely.

Limited information – best and worst case scenarios

* The patient may have a large upper gastrointestinal bleed, or may be severely hypovolaemic from continuous vomiting. This may also render them at risk of aspiration from their own vomit.
* They may have mild food poisoning, with a single episode of mild vomiting.

Who does it affect?

(a) Patient: If they are hypovolaemic or bleeding, their life could be in immediate danger. Alternatively they may be suffering something much less severe.
(b) Team:
  * The receptionists.

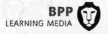

(c) Yourself: Potentially a time-consuming and stressful task.

(d) Other issues: None.

Using the MDT

If the patient is having a gastrointestinal bleed or something of similar severity, you will have to contact your GP colleagues for assistance. Again, you could call for help, and in particular try to enlist the assistance of someone with resuscitation skills. You could ask the receptionist to call an ambulance. On the other hand, if the patient is stable, you could ask the Practice Manager if they could help find a room to isolate the patient, and request one of the nurses or junior doctors to assess them.

Follow-up

If you delegate the assessment to a colleague, ask them to report back to you once management is initiated.

Recognising limitations

- Clinical acumen: Fully qualified GPs will have far more experience of dealing with acute situations in the practice setting, as well as managing risk. Colleagues who have recently attended life-support courses may be more up to date with airway and circulation management in that context.
- Time and workload: Although this task will use up valuable time, it is too serious to delegate from the start.

Comparing the tasks

Again, remember ABC in any acute situation. The airway could be at risk if the patient aspirates, and their circulation would be impaired if they were dehydrated or bleeding internally. This has been ranked first as it poses most risk to a patient.

Task D

The practice nurse would like you to see an asthmatic woman who she has put on a salbutamol nebuliser.

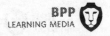

Limited information – best and worst case scenarios
- The patient may be a 'brittle' asthmatic who is experiencing a severe asthma attack.
- The patient may be experiencing a mild exacerbation.

Who does it affect?
(a) Patient: This depends on the severity of the attack.
(b) Team:
  - The Practice Nurse waiting for you.
  - The receptionists who are having to deal with the patients waiting to see the practice nurse.
(c) Yourself: This is another time consuming task.
(d) Other issues: None.

Using the MDT
If the patient is unstable you will need to request one of your seniors to help manage their condition and stabilise them. An ambulance will have to be arranged to transfer them to hospital, which the receptionists could help with. The receptionists could also liaise with patients waiting to see the Practice Nurse and explain the nature of the emergency.

Follow-up
If you leave the patient with the Practice Nurse you should go back and make sure that the patient is improving, and help arrange appropriate follow-up.

Recognising limitations
- Time and workload: manage by delegating to appropriate MDT members.
- Clinical expertise: as a junior trainee, you should seek advice from your trainer or any other senior GPs about any patient who is severely unwell.

Comparing the tasks
This task ranks lower than Task D because the patient is with a medical professional who has instituted management. It ranks above the other tasks because patient safety may be at risk.

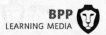

Task E

A patient with disseminated bowel cancer phones you from home asking for a prescription of painkillers.

Limited information – best and worst case scenarios

- The patient may be in excruciating pain without the painkiller.
- The patient may not be in any pain at all, but may want to ensure that they have enough medication to cover the weekend period.

Who does it affect?

(a) Patient: Depending on the above options.
(b) Team:
- The Pharmacist if they are required to dispense large amounts of a drug, particularly if it is a controlled drug such as opiates.
- Macmillan/Palliative care nurses if they are seeing the patient regularly.

(c) Yourself: Time consuming, logistically difficult task requiring extensive communication.
(d) Other issues:

Safe prescribing: It is generally inadvisable to prescribe large quantities of controlled drugs such as benzodiazepines, particularly if the patient has not been seen and assessed.

Palliative care: This branch of medicine requires skills in several areas, including communication, empathy, holistic medicine, and realistic practical decision making. The role of the MDT is extensive, and includes cancer nurses (or Clinical Nurse Specialists as they are referred to in some Trusts), social workers, counsellors, and sometimes even religious pastors. The GP and health professionals working in the community have a key role, as patients usually prefer to spend their final days in the comfort and dignity of their own homes with their loved ones. Patients can often be in agonising pain and discomfort. It is essential that their needs are not neglected, and should be given no less importance than acutely unwell patients. It is also emotionally demanding because the care is given over a long period of time, and often close professional

 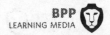

relationships are forged between patients and those involved in their care.

Using the MDT

Someone needs to talk to the patient and determine why they require the painkillers, and the patient's current status – a practice nurse or a GP who knows the patient well could do this. If a GP is conducting home visits close to the area where the patient lives, they could go and review him. A Macmillan nurse who sees the patient regularly would be the most ideal person to assess the patient, but may not be able to prescribe medication. If the drug is prescribed, you will need to liaise with the pharmacist before the pharmacy closes.

Follow-up

If you delegate the task you should find out what the outcome was, particularly if delegated to a nurse or someone junior. If it was a GP or someone senior to you, you may still find out for educational purposes and as a courtesy.

Recognising limitations

- Time and workload: This task will take a significant amount of time as it requires a thorough assessment of the need for painkillers, as well as liaising with the pharmacist and the palliative care team.
- Prescribing: The pharmacies may not be able to dispense large quantities of controlled medications, and you may not have much experience of prescribing controlled drugs.
- Clinical acumen: You may need the help of someone more experienced to assess the need for painkillers, such as a senior GP or an experienced Palliative care nurse.

Comparing the tasks

This ranks above Tasks A and B because it is related to a patient, and you may be able to delegate it quickly if the Palliative care team is involved. It ranks below the tasks C and D as there is no immediate danger to the patient's safety.

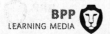

Task B

Your GP Trainer would like to go through your Personal Development Plan as part of your e-portfolio.

Limited information – best and worst case scenarios

- Your Personal Development Plan (PDP) may be long overdue, and the Foundation Programme supervisors may be on the verge of taking disciplinary action against you.
- This may be the only free slot your GP has to meet regarding your PDP.
- It may be the start of the academic year, and there may be plenty more opportunities to meet regarding this.

Who does it affect?

(a) Patient: There is no direct effect on patients, but on such a busy day you may be unable to undertake some patient related tasks if a lot of time is taken up formulating your PDP.

(b) Team:
- Your trainer may have designated this slot in his schedule and may have taken time out for this.

(c) Yourself: This task primarily relates to you. Important learning needs may be identified while formulating the PDP, as well as ways to address them. Your professional needs as per the Foundation Programme will also be fulfilled.

(d) Other issues:

Education and training vs. service provision: in a busy job, it can be all too easy to forget that you are a trainee whose role is to learn. Teaching and training is enshrined in the GMC's *Good Medical Practice* guidelines, and it is the duty of all doctors, particularly trainers, to ensure that a trainee's learning needs are identified and addressed. One of the main developments was the introduction of Personal Development Plans. The main aim being that the trainee and trainers could easily identify the trainee's learning needs, and decide how these could be addressed. This is vital not only for education, but also to ensure that trainees are practising safe and competent medicine.

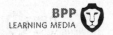

Using the MDT

Your PDP can only be completed by your trainer and yourself. If you have tasks that need completing you could delegate some of these to one of the GPs or Practice Nurses. Your trainer may be able to help you do this. The receptionists could inform any callers that you are busy and take messages for you.

Follow-up

If you do not deal with your PDP now, you will have to complete it at a later date.

Recognising limitations

• Time and workload: You have several tasks to do, and this one may not be urgent, but is certainly important.

Comparing the tasks

This ranks above Task B because your educational needs are important for you to progress professionally and practise competently. It ranks below the other tasks because it is not related to patient care.

Task A

There is a Drug Representative waiting to speak to you about a new form of simvastatin available on the market.

Limited information – best and worst case scenarios

• The drug rep may want to talk about an important new development in the prescribing of a drug.
• The drug rep may want to see you merely to meet you and build contacts in the local community.

Who does it affect?

(a) Patient: As important as the 'new development' may be, drug reps are not recognised as sources of evidence, and it is unlikely that their information will decisively alter your practice.
(b) Team:
   • The drug rep waiting for you.
(c) Yourself: This task will take up valuable time in a busy day.

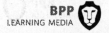

(d) Other issues:
Ethics: Different doctors have different views on how to deal with drug company representatives. Some GPs are against seeing drug representatives because they perceive them as mere sales representatives. They may feel that their information is biased, and they try to entice you with complimentary 'gifts' ranging from mugs through to international conferences in exotic locations. By accepting these it can be argued that you may feel compelled to prescribe their drugs. On the other hand, many GPs believe that drug representatives often publicise interesting and potentially important developments in the pharmaceutical industry of which doctors should be aware. They may argue that gifts are merely complementary, and that doctors are not forced to change their practice. There are no clear guidelines on this, and ultimately you will have to decide your stance in accordance with your beliefs, ethical codes, personal experiences and from your interactions with colleagues.

Using the MDT

Any other GPs in practice may be available and happy to see the drug rep instead of you. You could consider postponing your other jobs until you finish meeting the drug rep, and try to keep it as short as possible.

Follow-up

If you do not see the drug rep, you could reschedule the meeting for a time when you are less busy.

Recognising limitations

- Time and workload: You have several jobs to do – this task is by no means urgent.
- Practice policy: Your practice may have a policy which forbids you from meeting drug reps.

Comparing the tasks

This task ranks last because there is no immediate risk to a patient or anyone else, and will have minimal impact on your team and yourself.

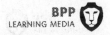

Suggested Answer for Scenario 4

(1) TASK C

I have ranked this as the most important task because the patient may be clinically unstable and have a life-threatening condition. I would immediately review the patient quickly to ascertain whether he is heamodynamically stable or not. If he was stable, I would consider delegating the task to a practice nurse, explaining the numerous jobs I had to do, and thanking her for her co-operation. If it seemed like a one-off and the patient was well otherwise, I would express empathy and reassure the patient that he will be seen as soon as possible, notifying the doctor whose list he was on about his episode of vomiting, and asking the receptionists to alert me if they had any further concerns. If he was unstable, I would ask my seniors to review him to give him the best possible acute care, and would also ask anyone with resuscitation skills to help if this was necessary. In this case, I would ask the receptionists to call an ambulance and reassure the patient that he would be taken to hospital very soon.

(2) TASK D

This task ranks above A, C and E because patient safety may be at immediate risk. Similar to the task before I will aim to carry out a quick assessment to diagnose the severity of the asthma. If it was severe, I would ask a GP to review the patient with a view to hospitalisation. In the meanwhile I would ask the receptionists to explain why the other patients were having to wait so long for the Practice Nurse, while I called an ambulance. If the asthma was mild, I would reassure the nurse that she was doing the right thing, offer to see the patient a bit later and help devise a management plan and follow-up for after the patient leaves. I would also show empathy towards the patient and the nurse as she must be very busy as well.

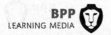

(3) TASK E

This task is more important that A or B because it relates to my patient, who is always my first priority, and I may be able to deal with it quickly by delegation. I would start by speaking to the patient over the phone and finding out why he needs more painkillers. If there is a straightforward reason such as the medications running out as per their designated duration of usage, I could simply print a prescription and post it to him. I may decide that I am unable to prescribe without clinically assessing him or her. As I have many jobs to do in limited time, I may delegate this by finding out if a palliative care/Macmillan nurse involved in the care of the patient could assess him, explaining my reasons for wanting her to do so, and reassuring her that she could contact me if necessary. Otherwise, a GP conducting home visits in the patient's vicinity may be able to visit if I provide them with detailed information about the patient's condition. If we decided that painkillers were not warranted, I would show empathy and sensitivity considering the patient's terminal condition, and identify other ways of making him comfortable.

(4) TASK B

This task is more important that B because I appreciate the importance of having a development plan and identifying my learning needs, not only to continue my professional development but also because it will make me a safer and more competent doctor. The effects of me delaying an important colleague such as my GP trainer are also significant. This ranks below the other tasks because there is no immediate risk to patient safety or care. I could formulate my PDP now, and ask my trainer to help me delegate my jobs so that this can happen without disturbance. I could also ask the receptionist to take a message from anyone who calls me asking them to ring back after the meeting. Otherwise, I could explain to my trainer that I have multiple tasks to do, and ask whether we could postpone the meeting, and apologise for the inconvenience caused.

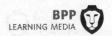

(5) TASK A

This task is ranked last because it does not affect patient safety, and will not render my colleagues or myself any major benefit. First, I will contact my trainer or Practice Manager to find out what the practice policy is with regards to drug-reps. If I am allowed to see them, I will explain that I am busy, and discuss whether we could postpone or shorten the meeting, while apologising for the inconvenience caused by this. I will then listen to them carefully and respectfully, and thank them for spending time doing this. I may also postpone any tasks which are less essential than this to a later date. If a GP is available and not busy, I would find out if they wish to see the drug-rep instead of me.

Reflection: What limitations in your own skills did you identify from this?

The most significant limitation that I identified was not being able to multitask. I was unable to find ways to articulate and express how I may have done this. In real life it is common to do more than one task simultaneously, especially when deluged with several problems which need to be addressed quickly. I also found it difficult to prioritise the task relating to my PDP. Although my natural instinct was to rank it low because it did not relate directly or immediately to patient care, it does have major long term implications for my own professional development. The long term benefits to patient care resulting from educational development of any form are easy to overlook when faced with several short term priorities. I found it difficult to maintain an overview of the long term situation during such a busy day.

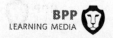

Practice Scenario 5

You are the medical SHO on-call in a busy city teaching hospital on a Friday evening. The hospital is very busy and there is currently a beds crisis, and you have two hours to go before your shift ends at 9pm.

Write the tasks in the order that you intend to rank them from 1 to 5, where 1 is the first task you would do, and 5 is the last. Write the letter of the task in the box provided. Justify your ranking and discuss any relevant issues relating to how you reached your decision. Write your answers within the box provided only.

At the start of the exercise you will be given five minutes to read the question, during which you will not be allowed to write. Following this you will have 20 minutes to complete your answers in the boxes provided.

(A) A nurse calls you from another ward asking you to review a patient who has a swollen red cannula site.

(B) The son of a patient on your ward starts shouting angrily at a nurse and kicks over a medication trolley.

(C) Your Registrar calls you from A&E asking you to help him insert a central venous line.

(D) The night SHO has just rung you on your mobile to say that he is off sick. He was due to start in two hours.

(E) You have to electronically submit your job application by 10pm tonight. Your shift finishes at 9pm.

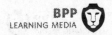

1.   TASK
2.   TASK
3.   TASK
4.   TASK
5.   TASK
Reflection: What would you do differently in the future?

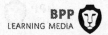

Suggested Approach to Scenario 5

Categorise the tasks:

- Definite immediate danger to life (I)
- Possible danger to life (P)
- Unlikely danger to life (U)

Task A

A nurse calls you from another ward asking you to review a patient who has a swollen red cannula site.

Although this is not an emergency, the patient may have a cannula-site infection, and may even be septic from this. His safety may be at risk if his condition worsens as a result of this. Hence this task can be categorised as a P.

Task B

The son of a patient on your ward starts shouting angrily at a nurse and kicks over a medication trolley.

The spillage of a medication trolley's contents involves serious risks. It may result in broken glass on the floor which could put both staff and patients at risk. If there was a sharps bin on the trolley, used needles may be exposed, putting people at risk of needle stick injuries and subsequent blood-borne infections. The perpetrator may do more damage or even attack people. There is immediate risk to the lives of patients, health professionals and anyone else on the ward. This is therefore categorised as an I.

Task C

Your Registrar calls you from A&E asking you to help him insert a central venous line.

Central venous line insertions are complex procedures, and used only with patients who have serious life-threatening conditions. However, your Registrar may be able to enlist help from someone else, particularly considering that he is in the A&E department. This would be categorised as a P.

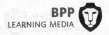

Task D

The night SHO has just rung you on your mobile to say that he is off sick. He was due to start in two hours.

There is no immediate risk to anyone's life here, but patient safety will be seriously compromised if there is no night medical SHO. As there is some time to sort this out, it would be reasonable to categorise this task as a P.

Task E

You have to electronically submit your job application by 10pm tonight. Your shift finishes at 9pm.

This does not affect anyone's safety directly as it is the 'personal' task. However it may be difficult to argue that it is emotionally distressing to such an extent that you could compromise patient safety. Hence, you could categorise this as U.

Categories and ranking:

Task A	P	Rank 2nd, 3rd or 4th
Task B	I	Rank 1st
Task C	P	Rank 2nd, 3rd or 4th
Task D	P	Rank 2nd, 3rd or 4th
Task E	U	Rank 5th

Task B

The son of a patient on your ward starts shouting angrily at a nurse and kicks over a medication trolley.

Limited information – best and worst case scenarios
- The patient's son may be angry, violent and completely out of control. He may be about to attack the nurse.
- The patient's son may not have intended to knock over the medication trolley, although as he is shouting he is still probably angry.

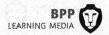

Who does it affect?

(a) Patient: The man may attack other patients on the ward, who are also at risk from any broken glass or needles from the trolley.

(b) Team:
   • Everyone on the ward is at risk.

(c) Yourself: You are at risk, but also need to deal with this crisis.

(d) Other issues: None.

Using the MDT

Anyone capable of restraining the patient would be useful, although ideally you would want the hospital security personnel present as they are trained to deal with such problems. Once the patient is restrained you should alert your seniors, in particular the Registrar on-call as well as the Clinical Site Managers.

Follow-up

You should reassure the nurse who has been shouted at, as they are probably in a state of shock and may feel afraid to carry on working. The ward sister or another senior nurse may be able to help you with this.

Recognising limitations

• Physical: do not try to be a hero. If physical restrain is necessary, either request as much help as you can, or call someone who is trained to do this.

Comparing the tasks

This is the first priority because the safety of everyone on the ward is at immediate risk.

Task D

The night SHO has just rung you on your mobile to say that he is off sick. He was due to start in two hours.

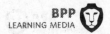

Limited information – best and worst case scenarios

- The absence of a medical SHO at night to review, assess or manage patients will compromise patient safety considerably. The rest of the team will become overstretched which could potentially end in serious error occurring.
- A replacement SHO may be found.

Who does it affect?

(a) Patient: This is self-explanatory. The lack of a vital doctor will mean that fundamental aspects of patient care will be compromised.

(b) Team:
- The rest of the night medical team (Registrar, FY1, etc) will have to work much harder, resulting in increased stress and fatigue. Their performance will be hindered as a result.
- Nursing staff would be affected by the remaining doctors being overstretched.
- The Consultant is ultimately responsible for the team, even in his absence. He may have to take practical steps to resolve the situation and liaise with the management team.

(c) Yourself: This is another time consuming task.

(d) Other issues:

Hospital management: it is important to know the structure of hospital management, and from whom to seek help. Obviously your own team and your immediate senior would be the first point of contact. There is usually a director or senior manager 'on-call' who can be contacted through the switchboard at any time if necessary. The Clinical Site Managers could also be helpful in such a situation to help co-ordinate the team in a way that minimises the impact of the SHO's absence.

Absence: There is usually a hospital policy to deal with absences, which should tell you exactly who to contact and how. It is vital for this to be done properly to ensure that absences are documented and systems for arranging cover can be implemented.

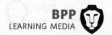

Using the MDT

You cannot solve this situation on your own, and your first point of contact should be the medical Registrar on-call. If you cannot get in touch with them, you could contact your Consultant, who would usually be the person responsible for liaising with the senior management team and directors. You could alert the nursing staff and your own team members about the crisis and see if they can help by working in a way that reduces workload for the night team.

Follow-up

There is no real follow-up involved in this task. You could offer the replacement SHO your phone number just in case they need further information about a patient you have seen earlier.

Recognising limitations

- Physical stress: you are approaching the end of a 12 hour shift and need sleep.
- Time and workload: you will need to spend some time to help resolve this problem.

Comparing the tasks

This task ranks below Task B because the impact on patient care is not immediate. It ranks above the other tasks because it could seriously compromise patient safety during the night.

Task C

Your Registrar calls you from A&E asking you to help him insert a central venous line.

Limited information – best and worst case scenarios

- The central venous line may be required urgently to stabilise the patient.
- There may be several nurses or SHOs in A&E who could help the Registrar. The central venous line may not even be required immediately.

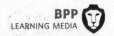

Who does it affect?

(a) Patient: They require a central line because they are severely unwell.

(b) Team:
- Your Registrar
- A&E staff: because the patient is currently in their department.

(c) Yourself: This will be a time consuming task, albeit not necessarily difficult if you are supervised by your Registrar. You will also lose valuable time that you could have spent completing your own tasks.

(d) Other issues: None.

Using the MDT

You could ask the Registrar to request another junior doctor or nurse in A&E assists them. The task could be delegated to your FY1, or if you decide to do it, you could delegate your ward tasks to the FY1. If the procedure is not urgent, you could offer to return later and help the Registrar.

Follow-up

If you delegate any tasks to the FY1 you should go back and find out if they have been able to complete their tasks.

Recognising limitations

- Time and workload: This task will take a significant amount of time.

Comparing the tasks

This ranks below B and D because the patient is with the Registrar in A&E where there are several doctors and nurses. It ranks above Task A because there are more serious implications for patient safety, and above Task E because it is has implications for patient safety.

Task A

A nurse calls you from another ward asking you to review a patient who has a swollen red cannula site.

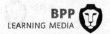

Limited information – best and worst case scenarios

- The patient may be acutely unwell due to a severe sepsis from the infected cannula site.
- The cannula may have become blocked, and may simply need to be replaced.

Who does it affect?

(a) Patient: The patient may be severely unwell, but even if there is a relatively minor problem such as the cannula being blocked, it will prevent the intravenous infusion from reaching the patient's circulation, and hinder their management.

(b) Team:
- Nursing staff: those who are administering the infusion.

(c) Yourself: Another time consuming task.

(d) Other issues: None.

Using the MDT

You could delegate this to your FY1 after talking to the nurse and ensuring the patient is stable. You could ask the nurse to remove or change the cannula.

Follow-up

You could ask the FY1 to report back to you if you delegate to him.

Recognising limitations

- Clinical acumen: if the patient is severely unwell you may need advice from your Registrar.

Comparing the tasks

This ranks above Task E because it is related to the patient. It ranks below the others because patient safety is not as acutely or severely compromised.

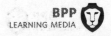

Task E

You have to electronically submit your job application by 10pm tonight. Your shift finishes at 9pm.

Limited information – best and worst case scenarios

- You may become unemployed as a result of a poor application.
- You will still get your first choice job despite completing a last minute application after the shift.

Who does it affect?

(a) Patient: Your patients will not be affected. It would be difficult to argue the impact of not doing the form is such that it will significantly hinder your performance at work.

(b) Team:
   - No effects.

(c) Yourself: Your employment, and hence your professional development.

(d) Other issues: None.

Using the MDT

It is unlikely that you will be able to utilise the MDT to any significant extent, unless you take time off in the shift to complete your application. Considering that the night SHO is off, it is unlikely that you will be able to find someone to cover you if you wanted to leave early to do your form.

Follow-up

None.

Recognising limitations

None.

Comparing the tasks

This task ranks last because there are no implications for patient safety.

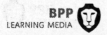

Suggested Answer for Scenario 5

(1) TASK B

I would deal with this task first as everyone on the ward including myself is immediately in danger. Unless there was a dramatic change in the son's behaviour, I would call security personnel immediately to help physically restrain him. If the son was moving to attack someone or cause further damage, I would briefly try to calm him down to diffuse the situation. If this failed I would shout for help and tentatively help physically restrain him - however I would try my best to avoid doing this as I am not trained in this and may thereby put myself in danger. Once the patient had calmed down or been restrained, I would try to reassure everyone on the ward, in particular the nurse who was shouted at, as she may be distressed and afraid. I would isolate the area where the trolley has fallen, as there may be broken glass or used needles putting people at risk of injury and infection. I would liaise with the ward sister and the hospital cleaners to help clear this. Later, I would talk to the patient whose son did this, and empathetically and sensitively explore his anxieties. I would also notify my Registrar and the Clinical Site Managers of the event, and complete a Significant Event Analysis form to learn from what happened.

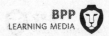

(2) TASK D

This task is important because the lack of a medical SHO will seriously compromise patient care during the night, more so than in C, E and A. I would be empathetic towards the SHO's sickness, although I would advise him to follow the hospital policy in order to report his absence. I would also contact my Registrar urgently and notify him about this, and offer to contact anyone else, such as the Consultant, if he was busy. Once this is done, I would make sure that I paid particular attention to minimising jobs for the night team. To help resolve the crisis I would offer to continue working for two hours after my shift. However, I would refrain from working longer, as I may be unsafe following such a long shift. I would also try to contact my friends and colleagues who are medical SHOs to see if they could cover the night shift. If a last minute replacement was found, I would do my utmost to provide a comprehensive handover with minimal jobs for them to do.

(3) TASK C

This ranks above A and E because the implications for patient safety are more urgent and significant. Only patients who are acutely unwell with basic physiological impairment require such invasive monitoring and treatment. However it would be very time consuming, and I may not be able to complete all my other tasks. I would explain this to my Registrar and suggest constructively that he ask a junior doctor or nurse in A&E, or even my own FY1. If this was not possible, I would ask if I could join him once my ward tasks were complete, or I would delegate it to my FY1, thanking him for his co-operation and offering to do some of his ward tasks later. I have ranked B and D above this because the patient is with a more senior doctor than me, and in a department which specialises in managing acutely unwell patients.

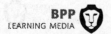

(4) TASK A

This task is important because there are possible implications for patient safety, as they may have a more severe cause or effect of redness and swelling, eg they may have a sepsis secondary to a cannula site infection, or may be severely dehydrated due to the cannula being blocked. Considering I have many other jobs to do, I would obtain as much detail as possible over the phone, such as the vital signs etc, and determine whether or not the patient was stable. If they appeared severely unwell I would review them and initiate management, asking my Registrar for help if necessary, and would hand them over to the night team to review. If I thought they were stable, I could ask the nurse to remove the cannula, and politely ask my FY1 to review the patient, explaining that I had multiple ward tasks to do, and ask him to report back to me to update me on the patient. This task is less urgent than B, D and C because the implications for patient safety are not as immediate.

(5) TASK E

This task ranks last because it has no implications for my patients or my colleagues. It is obviously important for me to complete because my professional development and financial stability are dependent on my employment. There is no information on when the application procedure started, although it is likely that it was a quite a while ago. I will reflect upon this, and try to prevent it from happening in the future by ensuring that I do not leave applications until the last minute. I will go home and submit it in the little time provided.

There is also the possibility that the form is virtually complete, and all I need to do is submit it by email. If this is the case, I could log on to a computer at some point in the shift and do this as it will only take a few seconds.

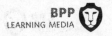

Reflection: What would you do differently in the future?

Through Task B of this exercise, I have identified crisis management as a learning need. I will address this, and find generic methods and strategies to help me deal with crises of any nature in any context. Other than this, I will also try to multitask, and do more than one task simultaneously. This is a difficult skill, but may be helpful, especially when initiating the management of any of the tasks or problems. I may also consider a different strategy, whereby I highlight the main points in all the tasks, and use these to prioritise them. This may be easier than looking at the scenarios as a whole.

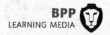

Practice Scenario 6

You are the Surgical SHO in a busy city teaching hospital on a Friday afternoon, while your Registrar is in theatre.

Write the tasks in the order that you intend to rank them from 1 to 5, where 1 is the first task you would do, and 5 is the last. Write the letter of the task in the box provided. Justify your ranking and discuss any relevant issues relating to how you reached your decision. Write your answers within the box provided only.

At the start of the exercise you will be given five minutes to read the question, during which you will not be allowed to write. Following this you will have 20 minutes to complete your answers in the boxes provided.

(A) One of the patients is concerned that he may have been given a drug which he feels is a contraindication to his condition.

(B) The Clinical Site Manager tells you that there are several warfarin doses to be prescribed in various wards.

(C) Your FY1 has arrived to do a Workplace Based Assessment under your supervision.

(D) A nurse bleeps you to review a patient who is short of breath who came out of theatre in the morning.

(E) A fellow SHO says that she wants a word with you in private, and seems tearful.

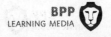

1. TASK
2. TASK
3. TASK
4. TASK
5. TASK
Reflection: What aspect of this exercise did you find the hardest and why?

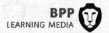

Key Issues – Practice Scenario 6

Issues around Task A

Use the information provided. The patient is well enough to express concern, which is a good sign. You may ask the nurse to collate information before you arrive, or delegate the task to your FY1, and reassure them that they can call you if needed. A major issue here is the demonstration of probity and professional integrity as per the NPS and the GMC *Good Medical Practice* guidelines. If the patient has received the wrong medication, explain this to him honestly, and apologise on behalf of the team. If he wants to complain the procedure for this should be explained to him. There are also system related issues – if the drug was contraindicated, was it not known to the nurses? If they did know, why did they administer it? And how did the doctor prescribe the medication? This requires a Significant Event Analysis to be completed to learn from the mistake and prevent it in future. Perhaps implementing an audit would also be helpful. This relates to maintaining high standards of patient care, as per the GMC guidelines. Above all, stop the drug and provide necessary treatment.

Issues around Task B

Warfarin is a very important drug which is only used for serious conditions such as pulmonary embolisms and atrial fibrillation. It is important to ensure that this task is completed. However you should use your time-prioritisation skills to decide where this can be ranked. The warfarin does not need to be administered immediately as it acts over a long period. You could demonstrate professional integrity skills by reassuring the Clinical Site Manager that you will do it as soon as there are no urgent tasks remaining. You could use your problem solving skills and be innovative, and negotiate a solution with the Clinical Site Manager to bring you the drug charts. If you are unable to do it, you could delegate the task to your FY1 or hand it over to the Night Team. Some of the warfarin dosing may be complex and you may need to recognise your limitations and ask your Registrar for advice.

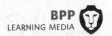

Issues around Task C

Teaching and training is one of the vital roles of a doctor as per the GMC *Good Medical Practice* guidelines. However, patient care is always your first priority, and if you have sick patients to manage you could apologise to the FY1 and postpone this. You could also reschedule it towards the end of your shift. If you decide to do it, you could ask the FY1 to prepare all the paperwork involved so that you can do it quickly.

Issues around Task D

You could talk to the nurse and find out how unwell the patient is. She may say that he is cheerfully talking to someone and his shortness of breath is intermittent. If so, you could ask her to collate vital information, and perhaps delegate the task to your FY1, asking him to report back to you. If the nurse gives an indication that he is acutely short of breath and unstable, you should see him and initiate management immediately as this may be a life-threatening emergency. You may recognise limitations in your ability to manage acutely unwell patients and may have to ask someone more senior to help you. You could also mention that you will show empathy to the patient.

Issues around Task E

This is important, not only for the empathy and sensitivity that you will have to show your colleague, but also because as an SHO, any problems she has may impact on her performance and subsequently patient care. You may need to help organise cover for her if she has to go, or perhaps help her with some of her work if there is a risk to patient safety resulting from the distress she is in. It would be insensitive for you to delegate this task, but you could consider asking someone else to hold your bleep while you talk to her.

Suggested order of ranking

D, A, E, B, C

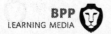

Practice Scenario 7

You are the medical SHO on-call in a DGH on the weekend. You have just completed the post-take ward round, and the consultant on-call has left. It has been a busy night, and there are a number of jobs pending.

Write the tasks in the order that you intend to rank them from 1 to 5, where 1 is the first task you would do, and 5 is the last. Write the letter of the task in the box provided. Justify your ranking and discuss any relevant issues relating to how you reached your decision. Write your answers within the box provided only.

At the start of the exercise you will be given five minutes to read the question, during which you will not be allowed to write. Following this you will have 20 minutes to complete your answers in the boxes provided.

(A) A patient had a cardiac arrest and unsuccessful resuscitation in the morning. His relatives have now arrived, unaware that he has died.

(B) Your sister who is at university has left a message telling you to ring her urgently.

(C) A ward nurse bleeps asking you to review a patient whose blood pressure is low.

(D) Your Consultant has called the ward and would like to discuss some patients with you tomorrow because he is going on holiday.

(E) The on-call pharmacist is on the phone, and would like to query the dose of a drug you have prescribed.

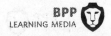

1. TASK

2. TASK

3. TASK

4. TASK

5. TASK

Reflection: What two things would you do differently in future?

Key Issues – Practice Scenario 7

Issues around Task A

This task does not have any patient safety implications, on which basis you could rank it lower than the tasks that do. However, there is a huge empathy component which is important when dealing with relatives as per the GMC *Good Medical Practice* guidelines. Your communication skills should be demonstrated as you explain the importance of breaking bad news and the way in which you do it. Obviously, you cannot have a comprehensive discussion on this, but basic points such as taking the relatives to a quiet private room and giving your bleep to someone else while doing this will score points. However, it is also a time consuming task, and you have many tasks to do, so you may decide to delegate it to someone else, preferably someone who was actually involved in the resuscitation and will be able to answer the relatives' questions in more detail. If you have time and space, you could briefly mention how you will arrange follow up with the patient's family, possibly through the bereavement services, which also play an important part of the MDT.

Issues around Task B

This is the personal task. Remember to recognise your emotional needs, and that the distress caused by such a phone call may hinder your patient care and compromise patient safety. It can also be dealt with very quickly if you make a quick phone call and find out that there is no serious issue. On this basis you could rank it first. If you are 'thick-skinned' you could carry with the other tasks and rank it last. Wherever you rank it, be explicit in your justification.

Issues around Task C

This may or may not be a clinical emergency, depending on the patient in question and how low their blood pressure is. An elderly lady who always has a borderline low blood pressure would be of less immediate concern than a young man who is suddenly faint and whose blood pressure has acutely dropped in the last few minutes. You could make a brief assessment over the phone by asking the nurse for more details, then delegate the

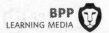

task to your FY1 reassuring him that he could ask you for help if needed. Alternatively, you could go and see the patient yourself and institute management depending on how unwell he is. If you feel out of your depth clinically, recognise your limitations and call for senior help.

Issues around Task D

This task relates to two major points. The first is making your patients your first priority, as the consultant may have some vital advice regarding their care. Second, you need to maintain good relationships with your colleagues as per the professional integrity part of the NPS. However, any acutely unwell patient needs to be dealt with first, and you may have to ask a nurse or ward clerk to take a message and tell the Consultant that you will call back later on in the evening. When you do this you could explain why this had to be the case, and apologise for any inconvenience caused.

Issues around Task E

This task relates mainly to patient safety and teamwork. You may have prescribed a potentially fatal dose of medication, or it may be a more routine query. The Pharmacist is an important member of the team, and the fact that they are waiting for you should signify its importance to them. You could rank it lower because it may be less urgent, as the drug will be withheld by the pharmacist until its administration is deemed safe. This could be completed quickly if you explain to the pharmacist that you are busy and that you will be late as a result.

Suggested order of ranking

C, E, B, A, D

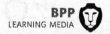

Practice Scenario 8

You are a GP FY2 in a busy inner-city practice on a Friday afternoon. Your surgery is running late, and there are a number of jobs to do be done before your antenatal clinic starts in two hours' time.

Write the tasks in the order that you intend to rank them from 1 to 5, where 1 is the first task you would do, and 5 is the last. Write the letter of the task in the box provided. Justify your ranking and discuss any relevant issues relating to how you reached your decision. Write your answers within the box provided only.

At the start of the exercise you will be given five minutes to read the question, during which you will not be allowed to write. Following this you will have 20 minutes to complete your answers in the boxes provided.

(A)   There is a rota for checking blood results which come back to the surgery. You are designated for this today.

(B)   You need to book tickets for a last minute family holiday, and the travel agent closes in half an hour.

(C)   One of your patients has phoned you asking for a repeat prescription of his diazepam saying that he has lost the pack prescribed two days ago.

(D)   The receptionists ring you saying that your next patient is having a nose-bleed.

(E)   A group of medical students attached to the surgery who you promised to conduct a teaching session for are waiting for you as scheduled.

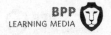

1.   TASK
2.   TASK
3.   TASK
4.   TASK
5.   TASK
Reflection: What were the key learning points for you from this exercise?

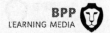

Key Issues – Practice Scenario 8

Issues around Task A

There are obviously significant implications for the patients whose blood results have come back, and there may even be life-threatening abnormalities such as hyperkalaemia or a very high INR. You could arguably postpone this task, as the blood tests may have been done routinely. Doing it after your antenatal clinic is unlikely to change the outcome for the patients, although delaying it until tomorrow may overburden you then. You could delegate part of this task (e.g. half of the blood results) to your trainer or any other GPs who are not busy after explaining the reason for this. If the blood results are severely abnormal and you find you need advice on the management of the patients, you may need to consult your seniors for advice.

Issues around Task B

This is a personal task, and you could rank it depending on how it would affect you and how you decide to deal with it. Holidays and other recreational activities are vital to avoid stress related burnout. The effects on your family will also be on your mind. If this task can be resolved with a quick phone call, you could justify ranking it high as it would put your mind at ease and make it easier for you to do your other tasks. On the other hand you could argue that it has nothing to do with your patients and you could rebook your holiday later.

Issues around Task C

This is a situation which GPs often find themselves in, particularly those who work within inner-city areas. The prescription of controlled drugs, in particular benzodiazepines, has caused serious problems for GPs and some have faced disciplinary action for inappropriate prescribing. Hence, it would be sensible to talk to a senior or your trainer before you prescribe it. Requests for benzodiazepines should be treated with caution, and it is always advisable to assess a patient before prescribing. There are several risks associated with overdose and the illegal drug market, where benzodiazepines are often sold on the street. However, it is important to empathise with the patient, as they

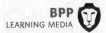

may have genuinely lost their medication, and may need it over the weekend. Many GPs in this situation would ask the patient to make a formal police complaint and provide documentation of the event if they were suspicious. Another option is to prescribe a very small amount – perhaps enough for the two days over the weekend, and then review the patient on Monday. This would provide a good demonstration of your problem solving skills, as well as your ability to think around issues.

Issues around Task D

Severe epistaxis is a clinical emergency, and until you assess the patient you cannot rule out this possibility. If it is, the patient will need to be stabilised immediately, and it is very likely that you will need senior help both for expertise and manpower. If the patient needs to be hospitalised, you could ask the receptionists to call an ambulance. This is always a difficult situation when you have patients waiting to be seen, particularly in the GP setting where you only have 10–15 minutes allocated per patient. You could demonstrate both your problem solving and communication skills by notifying the remaining patients that there will be a delay, explaining the reason for this, while asking another GP to add some of your patients to their list. If the patient is having a small nose-bleed, you could ask someone such as the practice nurse to help them and you can see the patient as per their agreed slot. Thanking the receptionists for their concern will demonstrate many of the professional integrity requirements.

Issues around Task E

Teaching and training is important, as is the need to maintain good relations among the team, including students. However, it is an unexpectedly busy day, and considering that there are patients who are acutely unwell it would be reasonable to reschedule the teaching session to a later date. Considering the pressure you are under, it is unlikely that you will be able to give the students your undivided attention while teaching them. Prioritisation is a key skill in medicine, and your students may benefit from the experience by observing first hand the pressures of a busy day in General Practice, and learning from this. This is also why explaining the reasons for rescheduling the session are important. You could consider

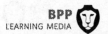

delegating the session to a colleague, although it is unlikely that they will have prepared anything for this.

Suggested order of ranking

D, C, B, A, E

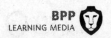

Practice Scenario 9

You are an A&E SHO in a busy District General Hospital on a 12pm to 12am shift in the 'Majors' section. The department is very busy, there is a beds crisis in the hospital and you have many tasks to complete.

Write the tasks in the order that you intend to rank them from 1 to 5, where 1 is the first task you would do, and 5 is the last. Write the letter of the task in the box provided. Justify your ranking and discuss any relevant issues relating to how you reached your decision. Write your answers within the box provided only.

At the start of the exercise you will be given five minutes to read the question, during which you will not be allowed to write. Following this you will have 20 minutes to complete your answers in the boxes provided.

(A) There is a call on the tannoy system asking for a doctor to go to the resuscitation room immediately.

(B) You have five missed calls from your wife on your mobile phone.

(C) The nurse asks you to review a patient who has chest pain. You have already clerked and referred him to the medical SHO on-call in A&E.

(D) A generic A&E teaching session for SHOs is due to start in ten minutes.

(E) A medical FY1 would like you to check a chest X-ray of a patient he has clerked.

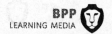

1. TASK

2. TASK

3. TASK

4. TASK

5. TASK

Reflection: If you could do one thing differently what would you do?

BPP
LEARNING MEDIA

Key Issues – Practice Scenario 9

Issues around Task A

The resuscitation room is where the most unstable patients are managed, and if someone is asking for a doctor immediately, it is very likely that there is a clinical emergency. You should go there immediately and at least find out the reason for the call. If there is a patient who is very unstable, you will need to initiate basic management, and will probably need your seniors to provide their expertise. You may even need to put out a cardiac arrest call or a trauma call depending on the nature of the emergency. If you feel you can manage the patient, you should do so, but if they are stable then you may want to explain to the nurse that you are busy and suggest they call someone else in a courteous and constructive way. You could help them by going back to Majors and asking one of your colleagues to help the nurse.

Issues around Task B

The personal task can be ranked anywhere depending on the impact it has on you. For example, you may be quite used to your wife giving you missed calls for relatively trivial reasons, in which case you could get back to her later on. Make full use of the facilities you have – you could text her asking her what the issue is, or perhaps give her a quick call to rule out anything serious and reassure her that you will ring back later on. If you need to talk to her at length, you could notify one of your colleagues such as your Registrar or Consultant, or perhaps even take your designated break period right now. If a serious problem emerges which will distract you and subsequently compromise patient safety, it is important that you recognise your limitations. You could talk to your seniors and consider leaving, possibly after helping arrange cover, or at least provide a good handover so that your colleagues can carry on after you leave. Apologising and thanking your colleague will demonstrate good communication skills, teamwork and sensitive use of language.

Issues around Task C

This may also be a clinical emergency which allows you to rank it highly. However you have already clerked the patient and

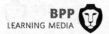

presumably initiated management, which makes it unlikely that there has been a new deterioration. You could briefly review the patient, ensure he is stable, and then wait for the medical SHO on-call in A&E to review the patient. If the medical SHO is busy, (which is likely considering the beds crisis in the hospital) you could review the patient yourself. If the patient has deteriorated and you feel out of your depth, you may have to ask your Registrar, or the medical Registrar on-call to advise you on how to proceed with management. If you are in the middle of a task you could explain this to the nurse and ask her if she could find someone else to review the patient.

Issues around Task D

Teaching and training are enshrined in the GMC's *Good Medical Practice* guidelines. Furthering your education is vital not only for your professional development but also to improve your clinical care and thus enhance patient safety. However, it is a busy day, and if you have ill patients who require your attention it may be reasonable to deprioritise this. You could ask your seniors for advice and whether they can help delegate your tasks while you are in the teaching session. You could apologise to the tutor and find out if you could obtain handouts or other useful learning resources related to the session. If there is going to be a poor turnout at the session due to the department being busy, you could suggest that the teaching session be postponed for another date, explaining the reasons for this and expressing appreciation that the tutor has taken time out to deliver the teaching session.

Issues around Task E

There are important issues related to teamwork, patient safety, and perhaps even teaching and training in this task. All trainees should feel that they have adequate senior support, and it is your duty to ensure that you receive and provide this in accordance with your designated roles and responsibilities. The patient in question may have a serious chest problem that requires immediate intervention, such as a pneumothorax. You could review the X-ray if you feel that this will not take you very long to do, and discuss it with the FY1. If you are in the middle of a task, or have too many other jobs to do, you could consider delegating it to another A&E SHO. If not, you could offer the FY1 an apology, explain your situation,

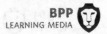

and perhaps suggest that he asks someone from the medical team or another A&E doctor. If you find that there is an acute problem with the patient, you may want to ask one of your seniors or the medical Registrar to review the chest X-ray and advise on how to manage the patient.

Suggested order of ranking

A, C, B, E, D

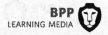

Practice Scenario 10

You are a surgical SHO, and are doing the morning ward-round with your FY1 while your Registrar is in clinic. The following tasks emerge during the ward-round.

Write the tasks in the order that you intend to rank them from 1 to 5, where 1 is the first task you would do, and 5 is the last. Write the letter of the task in the box provided. Justify your ranking and discuss any relevant issues relating to how you reached your decision. Write your answers within the box provided only.

At the start of the exercise you will be given five minutes to read the question, during which you will not be allowed to write. Following this you will have 20 minutes to complete your answers in the boxes provided.

(A) The Registrar would like you to assist him in theatre with an operation.

(B) A nurse tells you that a post-operative patient has a low urine output.

(C) The surgical SHO on-call in the evening has called in sick and medical staffing are looking for someone to cover for her.

(D) A patient whose elective cholecystectomy has been cancelled and delayed until two days later wishes to self-discharge.

(E) The ward-clerk tells you that the discharge Pharmacist called to discuss with you a query relating to a patient's discharge medication.

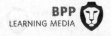

1. TASK
2. TASK
3. TASK
4. TASK
5. TASK
Reflection: What were the easiest and hardest aspects of this exercise?

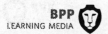

Key Issues – Practice Scenario 10

Issues around Task A

This task has implications for teamwork and patient care. It is imperative that you maintain good working relationships with your colleagues, and helping the Registrar is part of this. It also affects the patient who is having the surgery, as your help may help speed up the operation. However, you are doing the morning ward round with an FY1, and the safety of your ward patients is important. The FY1 may not be able to conduct a ward round alone, and may make unsafe decisions without you. We do not know their level of experience and clinical acumen. You may be able to let them do the ward round alone if there are no patients who are very unwell, and reassure them that they could contact you in theatre, and that you will return after the theatre list to catch up on the mornings events. On the other hand, if there are many patients who are unwell on the ward, you could explain this to the Registrar and suggest constructively that he finds someone else. Other options include joining the Registrar after the ward round, or asking your FY1 to join the Registrar in theatre instead of you.

Issues around Task B

The nurse is a key part of the team, and allaying their concerns is vital to maintain good relations within the MDT. Your initial concern should be to determine if the patient is acutely unwell. You could do this by asking the nurse for information which will give you an indication of this, such as the observations, and then prioritising the patient accordingly. If the patient is fairly stable, you could reassure the nurse that you will review the urine output once you reach them on your ward round. If the patient is unwell, you could see them next, and if they are acutely unstable (e.g. if they are severely dehydrated and on the verge of collapsing) you could abort what you are doing and review the patient immediately. If the latter is the case, you may have to seek advice from a senior on how best to manage the patient, and possibly liaise with seniors from other relevant specialties, such as medicine and ITU.

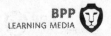

Issues around Task C

The on-call surgical SHO is pivotal in maintaining patient safety during the out of hours period. Their absence is a very serious matter and needs to be addressed as soon as possible. There are many ways in which you could help sort out this problem and assist your team. If you are free this evening, and wouldn't mind working extra hours, you could offer to replace them. On the other hand if you have something planned in the evening and do not wish to work then you could politely refuse but still do everything in your means to help find a replacement. This could involve announcing the problem to your SHO colleagues using every resource at your disposal, such as text message, ringing and verbally talking to them. You could also offer to stay for a little longer after your shift, and try your best to minimise the number of tasks to hand over to the on-call team. However, you are also doing your ward round, and may be dealing with some acutely unwell patients. As there is still some time to go before the evening shift starts, you could do all of this after your ward round finishes.

Issues around Task D

The key themes here are empathy, communication and problem solving. You need to explore the reasons for the patient wanting to discharge. They may be annoyed because they feel their condition has been devalued, in which case you may have to find out why their operation was cancelled and explain this to them. Patients can often be quite sympathetic towards the limitations that doctors may have. They may appreciate that a more acute case was prioritised above them, while feeling reassured that if they ever became acute they would also be given priority. On the other hand, the patient may simply have to go back to work, or may have children at home to attend to. You could express empathy and try to help them with their problem, perhaps with the help of a social worker if appropriate. If the patient is adamant on leaving, you could try to negotiate a compromise solution, perhaps urging them to call the hospital if they feel they are deteriorating or to return at a mutually agreed time.

Issues around Task E

This task deals with important issues relating to teamwork, patient safety, and even management. Maintaining a good working

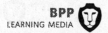

relationship with the Pharmacist is paramount for doctors in both primary and secondary care. Other than this, the pharmacist may make a suggestion that improves patient care, such as pointing out an incorrect prescription that may have potentially fatal effects on the patient. If the issue is not resolved you may not be able to discharge the patient, and this would worsen the bed situation, which would not only affect the hospital managers and discharge planners, but in the grand scheme of things also deprive an acute surgical bed to patient who may need it. It is also worth bearing in mind that every bed costs several hundred pounds per night – hence it is vital that the limited resources of the NHS are rationed sensibly and effectively. You could justify speaking to the pharmacist immediately, as the problem may be resolved over the phone within a few minutes. If you are in the middle of a task, you could ask the ward clerk to take a message from the pharmacist, and then ring them back after the ward round is complete. Remember to thank your team members for their assistance, and be polite and courteous to them – all part of good communication skills.

Suggested order of ranking

B, E, D, A, C

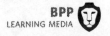

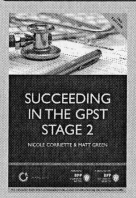
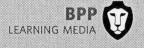

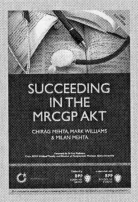
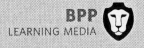

More titles in the MediPass Series

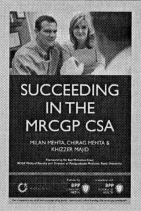

Do you want to pass the CSA exam first time and with a high score? Are you looking for a comprehensive CSA revision book?

Succeeding in the MRCGP Clinical Skills Assessment (CSA) is an essential part of progressing through general practice specialty training. This comprehensive revision guide is the most up-to-date available and contains a variety cases of covering the entire breadth of the RCGP curriculum. Written by doctors who have successfully passed the MRCGP CSA exam, this book is packed with advice and tips, including guidance on topics that candidates consistently struggle with.

This comprehensive MRCGP CSA revision guide:

* Describes the writers' memories of their recent CSA exams together with general advice on how to best prepare for it in those last few weeks (and hours!) before the exam.

* Includes a variety of cases spanning across the entire RCGP curriculum.

* Offers detailed guidance for each case on how to get the most out of each consultation by maximising your consultation skills.

* Gives both instructions for role-players and candidates for each case.

* Equips candidates with a structured, generalised approach that can be applied to any CSA scenario that may arise.

* Provides two full mock CSA circuits (26 cases) which can be completed under timed conditions.

This engaging and easy to use guide will provide you with everything you need to know to fully prepare for all aspects of the CSA exam, and is an essential book for anyone serious in excelling in this exam.

£24.99
October 2011
Paperback
978-1-445379-53-1

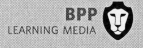

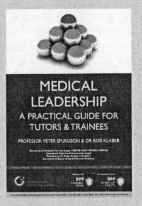
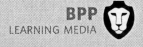

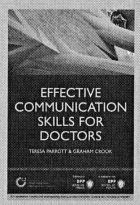
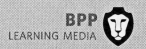

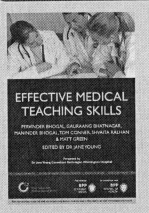
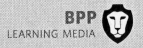

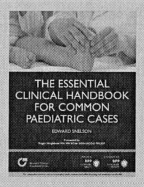
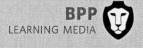

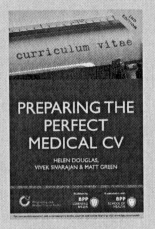
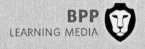

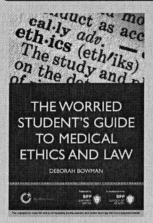

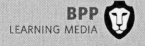